D1425112

THE HOSPITAL IN HISTORY

The hospital today is seen as the pinnacle of medical care, incorporating advanced machinery, devoted staff, and dedicated doctors, yet it is sometimes castigated as wasteful and interventionist. Even so the hospital has become central to the medical care of rich and poor alike, but this was not always the case. *The Hospital in History* casts light on what the hospital meant at different times and places over its history. Various historians have contributed essays which range from the medieval and Renaissance periods to the Enlightenment and the modern era, and from Europe to the USA. They examine not only the attitudes of patients and medical staff but also the culture and aims of those who paid for the hospital – whether governors or government. The authors look at the relationship between the hospital, state, church and society, the importance of philanthropists, the impact of industrialization and specialization, and the development of modern institutions.

These essays challenge traditional views in a field which is just beginning to be thoroughly explored, filling a large gap in our understanding of hospitals and the provision of health care in society over time.

THE WELLCOME INSTITUTE SERIES IN THE HISTORY OF MEDICINE

Edited by W.F. Bynum and Roy Porter,
The Wellcome Institute

Medical Fringe and Medical Orthodoxy, 1750–1850
W.F. Bynum and Roy Porter

Florence Nightingale and the Nursing Legacy
Monica Baly

Social Hygiene in Twentieth Century Britain
Greta Jones

Problems and Methods in the History of Medicine
Roy Porter and Andrew Wear

Vivisection in Historical Perspective
Nicolaas A. Rupke

Abortion in England, 1900–1967
Barbara Brookes

Women as Mothers in Pre-industrial England
Valerie Fildes

Birth Control in Germany, 1871–1933
James Woycke

The Charitable Imperative
Colin Jones

Medicine at the Courts of Europe, 1500–1837
Dr Vivian Nutton

Mad Tales from the Raj
Waltraud Ernst

THE HOSPITAL
IN HISTORY

Edited by Lindsay Granshaw and Roy Porter

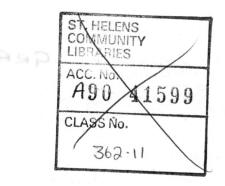

LONDON AND NEW YORK

First published 1989 by Routledge
11 New Fetter Lane, London EC4P 4EE
Reprinted 1989, 1990

First published in paperback by
Routledge, 1990

Simultaneously published in the USA and Canada
by Routledge
a division of Routledge, Chapman and Hall, Inc.
29 West 35th Street, New York, NY 10001

Filmset by Mayhew Typesetting, Bristol
Printed and bound in Great Britain by
Billings & Sons Limited, Worcester

British Library Cataloguing in Publication Data

The hospital in history. – (The Wellcome
    Institute series in the history of medicine)
    I. Hospitals, history
    I. Granshaw, Lindsay, *1954–*   II. Porter, Roy,
    1946–   III. Series
    362.1109

Library of Congress Cataloging in Publication Data

The hospital in history/edited by Lindsay Granshaw
    and Roy Porter.
    p. cm. – (Wellcome Institute series in the
    history of medicine)
    Bibliography: p.
    Includes index.
    1. Hospitals–History.   I. Granshaw, Lindsay, 1954–
    II. Porter, Roy, 1946–   .   III. Series.
    RA964.H67 1988
    362.1′1′09–dc19

88–18285 CIP

ISBN 0-415-00375-X
ISBN 0-415-05603-9 (pbk)

Contents

Contents

Contributors

Dr Martha Carlin received her PhD in medieval studies from the University of Toronto in 1984. The title of her thesis was *The Urban Development of Southwark, c. 1200 to 1550.* From 1984 to 1987 she was employed by the Institute of Historical Research, University of London, as research assistant to Dr Derek Keene, Director of The Social and Economic Study of Medieval London. Since July 1987 she has been the executive director of the new Medieval and Early Modern Data Bank at Rutgers University. Dr Carlin is one of the joint authors of *The Historic Towns Atlas*, Vol. III (London to 1520), ed. M.D. Lobel (Oxford University Press, 1988).

Sandra Cavallo took a degree at Turin University and then went on to postgraduate research at the universities of Lyon, Essex and the European University Institute. She has published a series of articles on family history and poor relief and is currently completing a comparative doctoral thesis on systems of charity at University College London. Her interest is in the application of social anthropological theory to seventeenth and eighteenth century history.

Dr Lindsay Granshaw is historian of modern medicine at the Wellcome Institute for the History of Medicine, London. Her PhD thesis was on St Thomas's Hospital in the nineteenth century and she is the author of *St Mark's Hospital: A Social History of a Specialist Hospital* (King's Fund Historical Series/Oxford University Press, 1985). She has published articles on the history of hospitals, specialized medicine, surgery, nursing, and nineteenth-century patients.

Dr John Henderson is Fellow of Wolfson College, Cambridge, and Wellcome Trust Fellow at the Wellcome Unit for the History of Medicine, University of Cambridge. He is currently writing a book on plague in sixteenth-century Florence.

Dr Caroline Murphy is currently the Education Officer (Essex) of the RSPCA. This work was carried out while she was a Wellcome Research Fellow at the Wellcome Unit for the History of Medicine, Manchester University. She received support from the Wellcome Trust for the completion of her PhD thesis in Manchester on history of radiotherapy of cancer in Britain.

Dr Roy Porter is senior lecturer in the social history of medicine at the Wellcome Institute, London, having previously been lecturer in European history at Cambridge University and Director of Studies in History at Churchill College, Cambridge. His research into the history of psychiatry was published as *Mind Forg'd Manacles* (Athlone Press, 1987) and *A Social History of Madness* (Weidenfeld & Nicolson, 1987).

Craig Rose graduated at the University of Bristol with a BA in history in 1985 and was awarded the University Prize in History. He has since been a research student at Selwyn College, Cambridge and is now in his third year of research on a PhD thesis entitled *Politics, Religion and Charity in London, 1680–1730*. He is currently a non-stipendiary research fellow of Selwyn College.

Dr Miri Rubin is a research fellow at the History Faculty and Girton College, Cambridge. She is the author of *Charity and Community in Medieval Cambridge* (Cambridge University Press, 1987) and of a number of studies on relief and mutual help in the middle ages. She is currently studying religion and ritual in medieval society.

Professor Dr med. Eduard Seidler studied medicine at Mainz, Paris, Hamburg, Heidelberg. He specialized in pediatrics in 1961, and took additional training in medical history 1963–7 (Heidelberg). He has been chairman and director of the Institut für Geschichte der Medizin der Albert–Ludwigs–Universität, Freiburg i. Br., since 1968. His fields of research are history of childhood, social history of medicine in the eighteenth and nineteenth centuries, history of nursing and hospitals, medical history in Germany 1918–45, and medical ethics.

Contributors

Professor Morris J. Vogel is Professor of History at Temple University in Philadelphia, Pennsylvania. His work in the social history of American medicine includes *The Invention of the Modern Hospital: Boston, 1870–1930* and *The Therapeutic Revolution: Essays in the Social History of Medicine*. He has also published in American urban and cultural history.

Introduction

Lindsay Granshaw

The sound of ambulances tearing through the streets bearing the very ill to hospital is common enough today. And few would doubt that the best place to be, if seriously ill, is in the hospital. The hospital is recognized as the central institution in medical care, for rich and poor.[1] It is often assumed that this was always the case. Yet until recent times, most people – especially if ill – would have endeavoured to stay out of hospital. Home was where the sick should be treated: hospitals were associated with pauperism and death.[2] How has this change of perception and use come about? Is there any continuity at all between the medieval and modern hospital, or does the very continuity of the name actually mislead? What is the hospital in history?

Hospitals over time have been much more varied than a casual glance at their present-day namesakes might indicate. Accounts of individual institutions have barely scratched the surface of their significance. Some valiant attempts have been made to record hospital histories, usually by those associated with them. Mostly written by doctors, they have tended to focus on the medical staff; it is sometimes difficult to detect that there actually were patients – or any staff besides doctors – in the institutions under scrutiny.[3] After long neglect, however, hospitals are at last receiving serious historical attention.[4] In recent years a general social critique has encouraged investigation of a range of institutions – prisons, schools, factories – and as the critique extended to medicine, the hospital, too, has become a focus of interest.[5] It is coming to be seen as an institution which, though central in modern times, need not necessarily be so, and has not necessarily been so. The hospital's function throughout history has not been constant.

A number of issues of importance are emerging from this new attention, but they are far from fully explored. The older histories tended to assume that hospitals were set up by philanthropic lay or churchmen according to the needs of the sick poor.[6] Patients would receive medical and nursing care before being returned home. In recent times, it is assumed, the hospital came to embody the best that modern medicine could offer – high technology, intensive care, and radical surgery.[7] Such assumptions are now under challenge. Historians are looking beyond the mere act of lay philanthropy and asking who gave, why they gave, and what their relationship to the hospital was. They are also trying, stretching sources as far as they will go, to assess who the patients were, what social class they came from, whether they were young, middle-aged, or old, whether they were friendless and without family, whether they were local or had travelled long distances for special treatment. Historians now want to know what patients suffered from, whether they were acutely ill or suffering from some slow, incurable malady, whether they were bed-ridden or mobile, institutionalized for a long time or a brief spell. Was the hospital simply a place in which to die, or did patients expect to return home either to continue their lives or for their last rites? On a more mundane level, what was the patients' experience of hospital – what did they eat, drink, do in hospital?[8]

The spotlight has also been turned on others associated with the hospital. If doctors were involved with the hospital – and it is no longer assumed that of necessity they were – what did the hospital mean to them? Were they actively and daily involved in care, or did they put in an appearance once a year? Was the hospital always important to the status of doctors – did they seek appointments or were they thrust on them, did they stay long at the hospital or attach themselves only briefly, did they teach or research in the hospital, did they announce proudly to the world that they held hospital positions, even long after they had ceased to practise there?[9] Where doctors are to be found, certainly in the later periods, historians concern themselves with the medicine on offer. Was it considered the best or the worst of the time? How does this reflect either the doctors' view of or use of the hospital? And, for that matter, that of the patient and the wider public? For some historians the clinic was 'born' in the French Revolution as the doctors' 'gaze' shifted from book learning to clinical experience. The hospital, as a result, was fundamentally changed, and later institutions show a total disjunction with their predecessors. Not surprisingly, this view has been challenged.[10]

Besides the doctors, other staff – from nurses to porters, from treasurers to chaplains – are now seen as important in the culture of the hospital.[11] Their social and geographical origins, their remuneration, expectations, length of service, their relationship to the patients and governors, the nature of their work, and the nature of their day, are all seen as part of the legitimate social history of the hospital. Placing hospitals in their social and geographic context, it can no longer be assumed that they were necessarily where the most needy poor were to be found, nor in the largest towns and cities, nor founded in response to epidemics. If their founding purpose was more to serve their endowers than the charity recipients, reasons other than the needs of the sick poor are likely to be paramount in determining such factors. For some historians, social control is a significant feature of hospitals, like other institutions. Were they part of an elaborate system of keeping the poor in their place, sweeping them off the streets and into the hospital, ensuring that they were speedily returned to work, or do other social reasons lie behind their foundation?[12]

In trying to answer some of these questions, wide varieties of sources can be used. Looking away from the published record of doctors – though never forgetting its use – there are the hospital records, the minute books, the records of rents, sales, and purchases, other financial accounts, patient records, from which valuable information can be distilled. Archaeological remains, town and monastic records, court proceedings, crown, state, and papal records, pictures, patients' diaries and letters, other literature, census returns, interviews – all can provide useful material on the history of hospitals. But as the authors here note, all sources, especially propagandist ones, have their difficulties as well as possibilities. Still, for all histories of hospitals, ingenuity in the use of sources is crucially important.

The essays in this volume, we hope, will help to open up

new lines in the history of hospitals – showing it other than dry institutional history, but rather as a microcosm of society. Most of the papers presented here were given at a seminar series at the Wellcome Institute.[13] There are a number of echoes between the papers, although the authors would not always agree with each other. The essays look at the position of the hospital in different societies, from medieval England to seventeenth-century Italy, from eighteenth-century Germany to modern-day America. No monolithic 'hospital' emerges.

A dominant theme that does appear is that hospitals served a major function for those who set them up and supported them, whether church or state, lay or medical; the founders helped to shape what the hospital was to become in each society. Thus, a doctor-centred approach to the history of hospitals is inadequate, but so too would be a patient-centred approach.[14]

The traditional concept of medieval hospitals is that they were founded by the church, more particularly by monasteries, and were outgrowths of hospices which accommodated pilgrims, the monastic sick, and possibly the sick from the surrounding area. It was part of monastic duty, laid down in the gospels, that care should be given to the sick and needy.[15] All these essays challenge accepted beliefs about the pattern of care, and notions of medieval institutions are questioned as much as any. Martha Carlin in 'Medieval English hospitals' (Chapter 1) explains that although medieval English hospitals or hospices certainly cared for the sick poor and for wayfarers, such strict definitions are misleading. There was a wide variety of hospitals, with a number actually finding the care of the sick an unwelcome burden which they later cast off. A point echoed by Miri Rubin (Chapter 2), Carlin argues that even if an institution did care for the ill, this did not mean professional practitioner care; she rarely finds evidence of a doctor giving assistance.

Lay endowment emerges as playing a major part in medieval hospitals, just as it did later. These were not simply monastic foundations. No doubt, as the well-off laity bought indulgences through large gifts to the church, they also saw hospitals as a way of ensuring that their account was in good order in the hereafter. Perhaps as important, they wished to be remembered on earth for their charity, and an institution was a concrete means of ensuring this. As a charitable act, it was the poor who were to be the recipients. Christian teaching dictated as much, and the theme of the rich giving to the poor through hospital endowment runs right through to the twentieth century.[16] Only those deserving of charity should be admitted: the disreputable should be kept out. A hospital gave its charity for the mutual benefit of giver and receiver; recipients therefore must be as deserving of charity as their benefactors were in need of giving it. In different times and different places this meant different things. Rubin argues, for example, that in Britain during the fourteenth-century plague, because the labour market was destabilized, with the poor misbehaving by moving to seek employment, the rich did not feel inclined to assist them through hospitals. Those who had formerly wished to support social order through philanthropy now found new reasons not to be philanthropic; not only were purse strings tighter, there was also a shift in the view of poverty as virtuous to seeing it as a source of disruption. The pursuit of benevolence as part of the social order was undermined and with it, she argues, late medieval hospitals. By contrast, John Henderson (Chapter 3) finds that in Florence during the plague years, more hospitals were set up for the suffering poor.

The close association of benefactor with benefaction is clearly revealed both in Carlin's paper and Rubin's. So dependent were the little institutions on their endowers – rather than, we take it, a more durable monastery – that many were very short-lived. Miri Rubin in 'Development and change in English hospitals: 1100–1500' (Chapter 2) finds instability built into the very foundations of these institutions of supposed 'perpetual memory' – they frequently died not long after their founders. Focusing on Cambridge and its environs, Rubin points out that rural care has received even less attention than urban care.[17] Stressing the varieties of caring institutions, Rubin suggests that the special characteristics of towns – whether they were a port, university town, or commercial centre – were significant in shaping their hospitals. The papers on the medieval and Renaissance hospitals show that those of us who study modern institutions should be wary of portraying earlier hospitals as peripheral to society. They may (or they may not) have been peripheral in overall health care, or they may be seen as peripheral to doctors – who were not that central themselves – but in other ways they were clearly of major importance. Hospitals played a far wider role than simply care of the sick. They provided social and religious rewards for the endower; they no doubt provided a service to those cared for, but they also acted in a variety of other ways. Whether in Cambridge or Florence, for example, hospitals could find themselves as part of a banking system. As Rubin argues, this, too, could be couched in religious terms, since it freed Christians from the hands of Jewish moneylenders.[18]

John Henderson in 'The hospitals of late-medieval and Renaissance Florence: a preliminary survey' (Chapter 3) finds a somewhat different pattern in fifteenth-century Florence, a much more highly-developed mercantile centre than any to be found in contemporary Britain. Not only were more hospitals set up in response to the plague – though Henderson does note, however, that attention turned particularly to orphans and widows, and only secondarily to the sick – but also there was more medical presence. While Carlin found little evidence of doctors in hospitals, Henderson finds active medical care in Florentine hospitals. Such institutions were not for the long-term ill, but for those suffering from acute illnesses, particularly fevers. Patients only remained in hospital on average about a fortnight.[19]

Florentine hospitals were widely admired not only for their practices but also for their architecture. As Henderson points out, the religious intent of such institutions was embodied in their design, which resembled churches, to the extent even of possessing altars and cloisters. The cruciform pattern emerging from Florence then pervaded the rest of the continent.[20] Florentine hospitals were clearly well-funded institutions with extensive property in both city and countryside. As elsewhere, both shady dealings and legitimate banking were to be found in them; widows for example, might receive a pension for life in return for pledging their property to the hospital.

Returning to Italy, but now in the Counter-Reformation period, Sandra Cavallo in 'Charity, power, and patronage in eighteenth-century Italian hospitals: the case of Turin' (Chapter 4) takes for granted that hospitals are more than simply about medical care. Italian historians have seen them, she argues, as pawns in church and state conflict.[21] The expansion of hospital provision in seventeenth- and eighteenth-century Italy has been seen as tied closely to the Counter Reformation, declining as Enlightenment 'anti-Christian' sentiments set in. But Cavallo sees the booming of hospital charity in Turin, for example, reflecting the climax of conflict between the court with its feudal apparatus and the new order of bureaucrats and merchants. The assistance of the poor by the better-off was only partly moral and economic. To a significant extent, she argues, it was to do with privilege among the poor themselves. Charities such as hospitals ensured the defence of the prestige and image of the social group to which the recipient of charity belonged. The emerging classes, as ever, invested in charity as reflections of their position. Hospitals were important to them, and bene-factors endowed beds not for curables, to be pushed through as rapidly as possible, so that hospital statistics looked good, but for incurables – often as an insurance policy for their elderly servants. The power to nominate people for beds was therefore significant.[22]

As seems to have been the case in Florence, doctors were already more involved in the Turin hospitals than in medieval and Renaissance institutions – before the university reforms which were supposed to have changed the scene.[23] Cavallo sees greater continuity in the hospital as a place of research, teaching, and medical practice than previous historians have done. Increase in medical teaching, though, resulted in yet another battle, between state officials and lay governors. Cavallo refutes the idea that change in the Turin hospitals was simply 'progress and rationalization' as the state took over: rather the substitution of an old élite by a new.

The role of the hospital in the wider political scene is the theme of Rose's paper 'Politics and the London Royal Hospitals, 1683–92' (Chapter 5) on late seventeenth-century London hospitals.[24] On the stage of St Thomas's was acted out in miniature all the political struggles of Restoration England. St Thomas's, like the other 'royal' hospitals, owed close allegiance both to its City masters and to its royal founders. In the last few years of Charles II's reign, through James II's, and into William and Mary's, St Thomas's found itself bound up in factional strife between Whigs and Tories. Rose suggests that the hospital, as a major property owner, dispenser of patronage, and a significant influence in South-wark, was not an institution which the Crown felt it could overlook. Charles II, supported by Tories, saw the removal of Whigs from important positions at St Thomas's as part of a wider attempt to remove Whigs from public life. However, from 1686, after James II's accession, it was the Tories who were under attack. Even the surgeons appointed at St Thomas's under Tory dominance eventually found themselves thrown out. It took the Whigs several years before they regained dominance; even then, the Crown, in the shape of William and Mary, sought to intervene again but, interestingly, then thought better of it.

Hospitals are also seen by Roy Porter in 'The gift relation: philanthropy and provincial hospitals in eighteenth-century England' (Chapter 6) as part of a wider pattern in eighteenth-century provincial England. He sees the voluntary hospital as an eighteenth-century invention to absorb charity. Using Braudel's notion of the gift relationship – he who gives, dominates – Porter argues that conspicuous, even self-congratulatory, philanthropy was the reason for so many infirmary creations around the country.[25] Hospitals served to close the rift between rich and poor – and here Porter identifies the chief patrons as being the aristocracy rather than the aspiring middle classes suggested by other authors. Infirmaries became the manifestations of civic pride over which even those of different religious persuasions could unite.[26] The system of annual donations tied in the benefactors closely; the voluntary hospitals did not go under as in medieval times.[27] However, as in earlier foundations, Porter sees the lay desire for a charity outlet rather than medical or patient need, or the professional ambitions of practitioners, as determining their establishment. Doctors offered their skills voluntarily because they too wished to demonstrate gentlemanly status through the gift relationship. In these hospitals, unlike those in Turin, it was beds for curables that were established. And, specifically, it was disapproved that servants of donors should be among the charity recipients. Patients were to be obedient and docile; no money should be taken from them, as that sullied the gift relationship.

In the modern papers several authors look at the relationship of special hospitals to society, as medicine itself became more specialized. Eduard Seidler in 'A historical survey of children's hospitals' (Chapter 7) asks what led to the establishment of sick children's hospitals, and what form and function they took. Unlike Cavallo, Seidler sees a real division between eighteenth-century hospitals and their predecessors. Hospitals change from homes of refuge to the *Krankenhaus* or institution for the sick. In earlier times the complex system of Christian charity was the locus of the hospital; by the eighteenth century the hospital was becoming medicalized, a centre for medical teaching, clinical research, and later the organization of healing for the welfare of all the population.[28] The earliest organized care for sick poor children (as children themselves apparently became the focus of greater attention) was dispensary care in their own homes.[29] Gradually this care was brought into the hospital, first in separate institutions and much later back into the general hospitals. Institutions in different countries seemed to vary and fluctuate (there was no single type) and the hospitals existed in flux between the self-interest of the medical profession and the needs of the sick child. In Seidler's account, therefore, lay philanthropy is already accorded a lesser role.

Picking up on the theme of the importance of hospitals to medical men in the last two centuries, my own paper ' "Fame and fortune by means of bricks and mortar": The medical profession and specialist hospitals, 1800–1948' (Chapter 8) looks at their relevance to medical specialization. Whereas previous foundations had largely been lay in origin, the nineteenth century saw the establishment of large numbers of small hospitals by medical men, as they sought a toe-hold in their profession.[30] Like the medieval hospitals, these hospitals were not firmly based and came and went according to their founders' interests and entrepreneurial abilities. It was the middle classes, not the aristocracy, who underpinned these institutions, as they bolstered their social status.[31] These special hospitals, it is argued, led the way in Britain to the much greater medicalization of all hospitals, with the accompanying breakdown of lay control. Assailed as unnecessary disruptions of the medical *status quo*, the special hospitals had nevertheless by the late nineteenth century become crucial to the medical élite; a large percentage of fellows of the Royal College of Surgeons, for example, had held an appointment with a special hospital by the turn of the century. Special hospitals played their part in the transformation of the image of the specialist from quack to consultant;

of the care for the sick in the home to care in an institution; from the doctor as peripheral in medical care of the majority to the doctor as central.[32]

A sense of coming full circle is gained from Caroline Murphy's 'From Friedenheim to hospice: a century of cancer hospitals' (Chapter 9). Here, in one area of medical care, the process is followed of establishing hospices to care for the sick with little expectation of cure, to the aggressive and interventionist high-technology and radical surgical cancer treatments of the first half of the twentieth century, but thence back to hospice care for the dying.[33] Here are nineteenth-century specialist hospitals along the lines of the others discussed in the previous article, but with a difference. They do not expect cures, good results, or to lure in philanthropic help on such a basis. Until, that is, the twentieth century radical cures – but then the patients for whom nothing can be done suddenly become an embarrassment. Murphy argues that, not surprisingly, given the direction of modern medical care, the cancer charities, the National Health Service, and the general hospitals remain remarkably oblivious to the needs of the dying, and it is again in the voluntary sector that such care is provided.

Morris Vogel in 'Managing medicine: creating a profession of hospital administration in the United States, 1895–1915' (Chapter 10) describes an important feature in the shift of the hospitals to centre stage. In America, as in Britain, the 'modernizing' hospitals, as they became the central institution in medical care, turned to professionalizing managers to run them. In Britain the image was of a civil servant or of an administrator trained in the army or empire, someone from the middle or even lower-middle classes who had risen through hard work and merit. In America the ideas of scientific management associated with Taylorism seem to pervade the hospital just as much as the industrial sector.[34] As ever, the hospital reflected the society which housed it. Many of the issues that the administration faced in the United States would be echoed in Europe: the need to forge a professional identity; the desire to combat the seemingly over-influential doctors; the need to run the institution efficiently. As the middle classes sought care in the hospital, the American administrators worried over curbing charity abuse without damaging potential fund-raising from paying patients.[35]

According to Vogel, it was third-party payment through insurance that shifted the balance of power away from the doctors to the administrators.[36] And in Britain that third-party payment – through the state – possibly had a similar effect. Certainly all blame overweening administrators for hospitals' financial crises. Perhaps hospitals should start their own banking systems once again.

All these papers bring out important themes in the history of hospitals, on a complex, broad scale. What emerges above all is that hospitals are the creation of particular societies. The interests they serve are not necessarily or primarily those of the patients. In many cases, especially before the nineteenth century, they were not those of the doctors either, but of those lay, state, or church leaders who established such institutions. By the time of the nineteenth and twentieth centuries, though, hospitals had become very much the objects of the medical profession, as commentators today usually assume they always were. These papers illustrate how that came to be and why that was not always so.

Notes

1. Any current political debate illustrates the perceived centrality of the hospital. It is seen as the workplace of the élite, and the place that patients increasingly choose to go directly to; see Brian Abel-Smith, 'Foreword', in Frank Honigsbaum, *The Division in British Medicine: A History of the Separation of General Practice From Hospital Care, 1911–1968* (Kogan Page, London, 1979), p. xiv. See W.G. Cannon, 'Hospitals in the UK', and E.C. Atwater, 'Hospitals in the USA', in John Walton, Paul B. Beeson, Ronald Bodley Scott (eds), *The Oxford Companion to Medicine* (Oxford University Press, Oxford, 1986), vol. 1, 551–65.
2. See for example, Florence Nightingale, *Notes on Hospitals*, 3rd edn (Longman, Green & Co., London, 1863); E.M. Sigsworth, 'Gateways to death? Medicine, hospitals and mortality, 1700–1820', in Peter Mathias (ed.), *Science and Society, 1600–1900*, (Cambridge University Press, Cambridge, 1972), 97–110; John Woodward, *To Do The Sick No Harm. A Study of the British Voluntary Hospital System to 1875* (Routledge & Kegan Paul, London, 1974); Henry Burdett, *Hospitals and Asylums of the World*, 4 vols (J. & A. Churchill, London, 1891–3); Morris J. Vogel, *The Invention of the Modern Hospital, Boston, 1870–1930* (Chicago University Press, Chicago, 1980).

3. See for example various histories of British institutions including C.T. Andrews, *The First Cornish Hospital* (pr. Wordens, Penzance, Cornwall, 1975); S.T. Anning, *The General Infirmary at Leeds. Vol. 1: The First Hundred Years 1767–1869* (E. & S. Livingstone, Edinburgh and London, 1963); H.C. Cameron, *Mr Guy's Hospital, 1726–1948* (Longmans, Green & Co., London, 1954); E.W. Dormer (ed.), *The Story of the Royal Berkshire Hospital 1837–1937* (Poynder Press, Reading, 1937); Sir P. Eade, *The Norfolk and Norwich Hospital 1770–1900* (Jarrold & Sons, London, 1900); A.G. Gibson, *The Radcliffe Infirmary* (Oxford University Press, London, 1926); Eric C.O. Jewesbury, *The Royal Northern Hospital 1856–1956* (H.K. Lewis & Co., London, 1956); O.V. Jones, *The Progress of Medicine* (Gomer, Llandysul, 1984); G. Munro Smith, *A History of the Bristol Royal Infirmary* (Arrowsmith, Bristol, 1917); J.B. Penfold, *The History of the Essex County Hospital, Colchester* (John B. Penfold, Colchester, 1984); P. Rhodes, *Doctor John Leake's Hospital* (Davis-Poynter, London, 1977). In P.M.G. Russell, *A History of the Exeter Hospitals 1170–1948* (pr. James Townsend & Sons, Exeter, 1976), Sir Derek Jakeway, Chairman of the Devon Area Health Authority, in the foreword describes the book as 'a disinterested labour of love'. In the same paragraph, this 'disinterested' author is noted to be consultant gynaecologist at the Royal Devon and Exeter Hospital, and in fact the first obstetrician to be appointed to the hospital!

For the United States see, for example, N.T. Bowditch, *A History of the Massachusetts General Hospital*, 2nd edn (The Hospital, Boston, 1872); A.M. Chesney, *The Johns Hopkins Hospital and the Johns Hopkins University School of Medicine*, 3 vols (Johns Hopkins University, Baltimore, 1943, 1958, 1963); J. Hirsch and B. Doherty, *The First Hundred Years of the Mount Sinai Hospital of New York* (Random House, New York, 1952); T.G. Morton, with F. Woodbury, *The History of the Pennsylvania Hospital 1751–1895* (Times Printing House, Philadelphia, 1895).

Many of the histories of hospitals by medical men are very useful, providing much information, even if they may lack a sense of overall context. Perhaps the best history of a British hospital by a medical man is A.E. Clark-Kennedy, *London Pride. The Story of a Voluntary Hospital* (Hutchinson Benham, London, 1979).

Occasionally a history has been written by another member of staff. See for example J. Gooch, *A History of Brighton General Hospital* (Phillimore, London, 1980). Janet Gooch is a nurse at the hospital. One of the histories of St Thomas's Hospital was written by its archivist – E.M. McInnes, *St Thomas' Hospital* (George Allen & Unwin, London, 1963). In the case of E.J.R. Burrough, *Unity in Diversity: The Short Life of the United Oxford Hospitals* (pr. Burgess & Son, for the author, Abingdon, 1978), the hospital administrator seems to have been inspired less by adulation of his institution than revenge against those with whom he worked.

Sometimes a local historian has been asked to write a history of a hospital or assist a doctor in doing so; see for example E.R. Frizelle and J.D. Martin, *The Leicester Royal Infirmary 1771–1971* (Leicester no. 1 Hospital Management Committee, Leicester, 1971). And occasionally a journalist has entered the fray. See for example J. Wilds, *Ochsner's. An Informal History of the South's Largest Private Medical Center* (Louisiana State University Press, Baton Rouge, 1985). Wilds has a keen journalistic eye for the wider setting of the hospital, is no great respecter of professional status (although he does regard medicine heroically) and ensures that the politics of the hospital come through clearly.

4. See, for example, M. Vogel, *The Invention of the Modern Hospital* (Chicago University Press, Chicago, 1980). Probably the most influential work in recent years has been by Charles Rosenberg, whose essays on American hospitals are now extended and incorporated into *The Care of Strangers. The Rise of America's Hospital System* (Basic Books, New York, 1987). For many years before the publication of this book, though, Rosenberg has influenced the study of the recent history of British and American hospitals. These influential articles include C.E. Rosenberg, 'The practice of medicine in New York a century ago', *Bulletin of the History of Medicine*, vol. 41 (1967), 223–53; 'Social class and medical care in nineteenth-century America: the rise and fall of the dispensary', *Journal of the History of Medicine*, vol. 29 (1974), 32–54; 'And heal the sick: the hospital and patient in 19th century America', *Journal of Social History*, vol. 10 (1977), 428–47; 'The therapeutic revolution. Medicine, meaning and social change in nineteenth-century America', *Perspectives in Biology and Medicine*, vol. 20 (1977), 485–506; 'Inward vision and outward glance: the shaping of the American hospital, 1880–1914', *Bulletin of the History of Medicine*, vol. 53 (1979), 346–91; 'Florence Nightingale on contagion: the hospital as moral universe', in C.E. Rosenberg (ed.), *Healing and History: Essays for George Rosen* (Science History Publications, New York, 1979), 116–36; 'From almshouse to hospital: the shaping of Philadelphia General Hospital', *Milbank Memorial Fund Quarterly*, vol. 60 (1982), 108–54; 'Disease and social order in America: perceptions and expectations', *Milbank Memorial Fund Quarterly*, vol. 64, supl. no. 1 (1986), 34–55.

Other American historians of hospitals include D. Rosner, *A Once Charitable Enterprise: Hospitals and Health Care in Brooklyn and New York, 1885–1915* (Cambridge University Press, Cambridge, 1982). R. Stevens, '"A poor sort of memory": voluntary hospitals and government before the great depression', *Health and Society*, vol. 60 (1982), 551–84; R. Stevens, 'Sweet charity: state aid to hospitals in Pennsylvania, 1870–1910', *Bulletin of the History of Medicine*, vol. 58 (1984), 287–314, 474–95; V.G. Drachman, *Hospital with a Heart. Women Doctors and the Paradox of Separatism at the New England Hospital, 1862–1969* (Cornell University Press, Ithaca and London, 1984).

Introduction

In Britain we have B. Abel-Smith's *The Hospitals 1880–1948. A Study in Social Administration in England and Wales* (Heinemann, London, 1964), a very useful overview of the past century and a half, but which explicitly addresses hospitals from an administrative point of view; F.N.L. Poynter (ed.), *The Evolution of Hospitals in Britain* (Pitman, London, 1968); also L. Granshaw, *St Mark's Hospital, London: A Social History of a Specialist Hospital* (King's Fund Historical Series/Oxford University Press, London, 1985); J.V. Pickstone, *Medicine and Industrial Society: A History of Hospital Development in Manchester and its Region, 1752–1946* (Manchester University Press, Manchester, 1985); G.B. Risse, *Hospital Life in Enlightenment Scotland. Care and Teaching at the Royal Infirmary of Edinburgh* (Cambridge University Press, Cambridge, London and New York, 1986). For other information on Scotland see D. Hamilton, *The Healers. A History of Medicine in Scotland* (Canongate, Edinburgh, 1981).

A number of dissertations have also been written; see for example S.G. Cherry, 'The role of the English provincial hospitals in the 18th and 19th Centuries', PhD thesis, University of East Anglia, 1977; L. Granshaw, 'St Thomas's Hospital, London, 1850–1900', PhD thesis, Bryn Mawr College, USA, 1981; J. Lynaugh, 'The community hospitals of Kansas City, Missouri, 1870–1915', PhD thesis, University of Kansas, 1982; J.M. Kingsdale, 'The growth of hospitals: an economic history in Baltimore', PhD thesis, University of Michigan, 1981; Susan Lawrence, 'Science and medicine at the London hospitals: the development of teaching and research, 1750–1815', PhD thesis, University of Toronto, 1985.

5. For critiques of institutions and of medicine, see I. Illich, *Deschooling Society* (Calder & Boyars, London, 1971); M. Foucault, *Discipline and Punish: The Birth of the Prison* (Peregrine, London, 1979); I. Illich, *Limits to Medicine* (Pelican, London, 1977); B. Inglis, *The Diseases of Civilisation* (Hodder & Stoughton, London, 1981); I. Kennedy, *The Unmasking of Medicine* (Allen & Unwin, London, 1981). For examples of essays on a range of Victorian social institutions, see H.J. Dyos and M. Wolff (eds), *The Victorian City: Image and Reality* (Routledge & Kegan Paul, London and Boston, 1973).

6. See for example C. Dainton, *The Story of England's Hospitals* (Museum Press, London, 1961).

7. S.J. Reiser, *Medicine and the Reign of Technology* (Cambridge University Press, Cambridge, London, and New York, 1978).

8. See Vogel, *The Invention of the Modern Hospital*; Granshaw, *St Mark's Hospital*; Rosenberg, *The Care of Strangers*.

9. W.F. Bynum, 'Physicians, hospitals and career structures in eighteenth century London', in W.F. Bynum and R. Porter (eds), *William Hunter and the Eighteenth-Century Medical World* (Cambridge University Press, Cambridge, 1985), 105–28; for professionalization, especially in medicine, see E. Freidson, *Profession of Medicine*

14

(Dodd, Mead, New York, 1970); E. Freidson, *Professional Powers. A Study of the Institutionalisation of Formal Knowledge* (University of Chicago Press, Chicago and London, 1986); N. Parry and J. Parry, *The Rise of the Medical Profession* (Croom Helm, London, 1976); M. Jeanne Peterson, *The Medical Profession in Mid-Victorian London* (University of California Press, Berkeley, California, 1978); I. Waddington, *The Medical Profession in the Industrial Revolution* (Gill & Macmillan, Dublin, 1984).

10. M. Foucault, *The Birth of the Clinic. An Archaeology of Medical Perception*, trans. A.M. Sheridan (Tavistock, London, 1976); E.H. Ackerknecht, *Medicine at the Paris Hospital, 1794–1848* (Johns Hopkins Press, Baltimore, 1967); Toby Gelfand, *Professionalizing Modern Medicine; Paris Surgeons and Medical Science and Institutions in the 18th century* (Greenwood Press, Westport, Conn., London, 1980).

11. C.E. Rosenberg, 'Inward vision and outward glance: the shaping of the American Hospital, 1880–1914', *Bulletin of the History of Medicine*, vol. 53 (1979), 346–91; Granshaw, 'St Thomas's Hospital'; for changing views on the history of nursing see C. Davies (ed.), *Rewriting Nursing History* (Croom Helm, London, 1980); C. Maggs, *The Origins of General Nursing* (Croom Helm, London, 1983); M.E. Baly, *Nursing and Social Change* (Heinemann, London, 1982); B. Abel-Smith, *A History of the Nursing Profession* (Heinemann, London, 1982); M.E. Baly, *Florence Nightingale and the Nursing Legacy* (Croom Helm, London, 1986).

12. See for example, Andrew Wear, 'Caring for the sick poor in St Bartholomew Exchange: 1580–1676', in W.F. Bynum (ed.), *Living and Dying in London* (Routledge, London, 1989).

13. Academic years 1986–7.

14. In history of medicine, as in social history, recent focus has been on the ordinary person. For history of medicine, that has meant looking at the patient or potential patient. For recent patient-centred history see R. Porter (ed.), *Patients and Practitioners: Lay Perceptions of Medicine in Pre-Industrial Society* (Cambridge University Press, Cambridge, 1985).

15. See for example, Dainton, *The Story of England's Hospitals*; C. Graves, *The Story of St Thomas's, 1106–1947* (pr. St Thomas's, dist. Faber & Faber, London, 1947); D. Knowles and R. Neville Hadcock, *Medieval Religious Houses, England and Wales* (Longman, London, 1971); R.M. Clay, *The Mediaeval Hospitals of England* (Methuen, London, 1909); Walter H. Godfrey, *The English Alms-house* (Faber & Faber, London, 1955); C. Rawcliffe, 'The hospitals of later medieval London', *Medical History*, vol. 28 (1984), 1–21.

16. It is instructive to compare with practice in other cultures; see Lawrence Conrad on medieval middle-eastern hospitals, L.I. Conrad and V. Nutton, *Jundishapur: From Myth to History* (Darwin Press, Princeton, forthcoming). However, Judaic, Christian, and Moslem cultures were closely interlinked, and therefore one system was likely to influence another.

17. In France the Annales school has attempted to tell the history of rural areas; see for example E. Le Roy Ladurie, *Montaillou: village occitan de 1294 à 1324* (Gallimard, Paris, 1976), based on Inquisition reports.

18. So too did other medieval institutions; Knowles and Hadcock, *Medieval Religious Houses*.

19. This was half the average time of at least one London hospital in the nineteenth century; see Granshaw, 'St Thomas's Hospital', p. 78.

20. For further information on the history of hospital architecture see J.D. Thompson and G. Goldin, *The Hospital: A Social and Architectural History* (Yale University Press, New Haven and London, 1975).

21. In much Italian history of church and state, conflict looms large; B.S. Pullan, *Rich and Poor in Renaissance Venice. The Social Institutions of a Catholic State to 1620* (Blackwell, Oxford, 1971).

22. For the nature of philanthropy in Britain see David Owen, *English Philanthropy 1660–1960* (Cambridge, Mass., Belknap Press, 1965). In eighteenth–century Britain it was not seen as appropriate to admit servants.

23. See Foucault, *The Birth of the Clinic*; Risse, *Hospital Life in Enlightenment Scotland*; and Johanna Geyer-Kordesch, 'German medical education in the eighteenth century: the Prussian context and its influence', in W.F. Bynum and R. Porter (eds), *William Hunter and the Eighteenth-Century Medical World* (Cambridge University Press, Cambridge, 1985), 177–206.

24. For further discussion of political dimensions see A. Wilson, 'The early history of the Westminster Hospital', unpublished paper given to the Wellcome Unit for the History of Medicine, University of Cambridge, October 1983.

25. R.H. Titmuss, *The Gift Relationship* (George Allen & Unwin, London, 1970).

26. Museums, parks, and libraries also benefited from this movement; see R.K. Webb, *Modern England From the Eighteenth Century to the Present* (Harper & Row, New York and London, 1968).

27. One of the chief features of the voluntary hospitals was their voluminous annual reports, which recorded lists of names of donors, including the amounts donated.

28. Geyer-Kordesch, 'German medical education'.

29. See Z. Cope, 'The history of the dispensary movement', in Poynter (ed.), *Evolution of Hospitals in Britain*; T. Hunt (ed.), *The Medical Society of London 1773–1973* (Heinemann, London, 1972); G.F. Still, *The History of Paediatrics* (Oxford University Press, London, 1931).

30. For the various methods of covertly 'advertising' see Peterson, *Medical Profession in Mid-Victorian London*.

31. See for example, William Taylor Copeland, Lord Mayor of London in 1835, whose father jointly formed the Copeland Spode

China Works and made a fortune, whereupon W.T. Copeland sought to establish himself in the social hierarchy, successfully in the City of London and less so through Parliament, where he was accused of all the sins of the *nouveau riche*. In his rise, he patronized a number of 'good works', including several hospitals; see Granshaw, *St Mark's Hospital*.

32. On the rise of specialization in medicine, see G. Rosen, *The Specialization of Medicine* (Froben Press, New York, 1944); R. Stevens, *Medical Practice in Modern England: The Impact of Specialisation and State Medicine* (Yale University Press, New Haven, 1966); R. Kershaw, *Special Hospitals* (George Putnam & Sons, London, 1909).

33. S. Stoddard, *The Hospice Movement* (Jonathan Cape, London, 1979).

34. For Taylor's scientific management see F.W. Taylor, 'A piece-work system', *Transactions of the American Society of Mechanical Engineers*, no. 16 (1895), 856–903. For commentary, see D.F. Noble, *America by Design: Science, Technology, and the Rise of Corporate Capitalism* (Knopf, New York, 1979); C.E. Rosenberg, 'Inward vision and outward glance: the shaping of the American Hospital, 1880–1914', *Bulletin of the History of Medicine* no. 53 (1979), 346–91. For Britain see Granshaw, 'St Thomas's Hospital', 48–59.

35. For concern about charity abuse, and the advocacy of paying patients, see Henry Burdett, *Hospitals and Asylums of the World*, 4 vols, 1891–3; Burdett, *Cottage Hospitals, General, Fever, and Convalescent. Their Progress, Management, and Work in Great Britain and Ireland, and the United States of America*, 3rd edn (The Scientific Press, London, 1896) 1; D. Rosner, *A Once Charitable Enterprise: Hospitals and Health Care in Brooklyn and New York, 1885–1915* (Cambridge University Press, Cambridge, 1982).

36. For further information see R. Stevens, *Medical Practice in Modern England: The Impact of Specialisation and State Medicine* (Yale University Press, New Haven, 1966); R. Stevens, *American Medicine and the Public Interest* (Yale University Press, New Haven, 1971); D.M. Fox, *Health Policies, Health Politics: The British and American Experience, 1911–1965* (Princeton University Press, Princeton, 1986); R. Levitt, *The Reorganised National Health Service* (Croom Helm, London, 1979). For Great Britain see R. Hodgkinson, *The Origins of the National Health Service: The Medical Service* (Wellcome Institute, London, 1967); D. Fraser, *The Evolution of the British Welfare State* (Macmillan, London, 1984); J. Pater, *The Origins of the National Health Service* (King's Fund Historical Series, London, 1981); C. Webster, *The Health Services Since the War. Volume 1. Problems of Health Care: The National Health Service Before 1957* (HMSO, London, 1988). On American insurance, see Ronald L. Numbers, 'The third party: health insurance in America', in Vogel and Rosenberg (eds), *The Therapeutic Revolution*, 177–200.

I

Medieval

1

Medieval English hospitals

Martha Carlin

The medieval term 'hospital', *hospitale* in Latin, embraced four main types of institution: leper houses, almshouses, hospices for poor wayfarers and pilgrims, and institutions that cared for the sick poor. There is as yet no satisfactory general study of medieval English hospitals. The most useful work to date is David Knowles' and Neville Hadcock's *Medieval Religious Houses, England and Wales* (2nd edition, 1971), which contains a gazetteer of some 1,103 hospitals, with a brief history of each.[1] These histories were compiled by the authors from printed sources, particularly Dugdale's *Monasticon Anglicanum* (1817–30 edition), Tanner's *Notitia Monastica* (1744 edition), and the *Victoria County Histories*.

Another source frequently cited by Knowles and Hadcock is R.M. Clay's *The Medieval Hospitals of England* (1909). This book, however, is seriously flawed by meagre documentation and by the author's romantic and essentially unscholarly treatment of the subject. Clay's intention was, through this study, 'to secure a fuller recognition of the widespread activity of the Church of England in former days'. She saw the numerous hospital foundations as predominantly ecclesiastical in character, charitable and pious in tone, and stable and effective in activity, from their origins until the Dissolution, when 'charity was crippled for a time by the confiscation of endowments designed for the relief of the destitute, until a new generation of philanthropists arose and endeavored to replace them'.[2]

In contrast was the view of Margaret Seymour in an unpublished King's College, London, MA thesis (1947) on 'The organisation, personnel and functions of the medieval hospital in the later middle ages'. This thesis was handicapped, as the author acknowledged, by the wartime and immediately postwar unavailability of most manuscript sources. Nevertheless, it is a useful study, based on the printed sources then available, and concentrating particularly on the administrative history of medieval English hospitals. Because of this focus, however, the author tended to lump together all types of hospital as being united by their shared administrative characteristics. This enabled her to demonstrate her main thesis, that in all classes of hospital decay and decline were rife in the later medieval period, principally because of financial maladministration. It does, however, make her work rather difficult to use for anyone studying either a particular type of hospital, or individual hospitals, with the exception of St Leonard's, York, to whose history she paid special attention.

Among the most useful primary sources in print are the *Valor Ecclesiasticus* and the *Calendars* of the Patent Rolls, Close Rolls, Inquisitions Miscellaneous, and Papal Letters. Episcopal registers, some of which have been printed, are another important source, particularly of foundation records and visitation reports. For example, the text of the original foundation charter of the hospital of St Thomas the Martyr, Southwark, which is generally assumed to have been lost, survives in a transcript made in the early fourteenth century in the register of John de Stratford, Bishop of Winchester.[3] In the case of hospitals of which the monarch was patron, such records are included among the Chancery Miscellanea, which are partially printed in the *Calendar of Inquisitions Miscellaneous*. Wills, many of which are printed or calendared, also provide much information on hospitals and on the popular support of them.

Of the four classes of hospital described at the beginning of this paper, the first and perhaps the easiest to distinguish is the leper hospital. Of the 1,103 hospitals in England and Wales listed by Knowles and Hadcock, some 345 (31 per cent) were intended wholly or in part for lepers. Leper hospitals generally had the most strictly-defined function among the medieval hospitals. Their inmates were required to be segregated for life from the rest of the population, to wear a distinctive and enveloping form of dress, and to refrain from casual as well as long-term contact with the healthy. Leper hospitals, whose inmates included both religious and lay persons of both sexes, were among the earliest hospitals to be founded in England. Of those leper hospitals whose foundation dates are known, the majority were founded between 1084 and 1224, although there were some later foundations and re-foundations. The later foundations included the hospital at Little Torrington in Devon (1344), and the hospitals of St Leonard, Sudbury (1372), and St John the Evangelist, Thetford (1387), while Holy Innocents, Lincoln, was re-founded in 1461 as an almshouse with accommodation for three lepers.[4] Leper hospitals commonly were placed on the outskirts of towns, to which entry was forbidden to lepers. Most leper hospitals were small, with perhaps fewer than a dozen inmates, although there were some larger houses. The hospital at Sherburn, Durham, for example, was founded *c.* 1181 to house sixty-five leprous monks, nuns, and other religious from monasteries in the north of England.[5] Most leper hospitals were intended to care for lepers only, although a number did accommodate or come to accommodate other inmates as well, usually almspersons.

Most leper hospitals had become redundant by the mid-fifteenth century, and many, particularly the small and poorly endowed, also had become derelict by that time.[6] Those that survived were often re-founded or reconstituted as almshouses, or in some cases as colleges of secular canons, chantry chapels, or grammar schools. The leper hospital at Sherburn, for example, which had been founded for a master, three priests, and sixty-five lepers, had become impoverished by 1429. It was reconstituted in 1434 for a master, four chaplains, four clerks, two boy choristers, two lepers if so many could be found, and thirteen poor brothers, with a woman servant to look after them.[7] The leper hospital of St Giles, Holborn (London), founded in 1101 for forty lepers, was housing nine lepers in 1402, and fourteen paupers in 1535.[8]

Almshouses formed the second and most numerous of the four classes of hospitals. Of Knowles and Hadcock's 1,103 hospitals, some 742 (67 per cent) are listed as almshouses or as having included almspeople among their inmates. Almshouses fell into two broad sub-categories: those intended for the poor in general; and those to which admission was restricted, as, for example, to local residents or to members of the founder's guild or fraternity. Most almshouses received male inmates only, although some were intended solely for women. A number took in poor persons of both sexes, although in such cases the men and women were strictly segregated within the hospital, even if they were married.

Neither leper hospitals nor almshouses provided medical care as such. The inmates were expected to lead a semi-monastic life, typically eating and sleeping in common halls, wearing a distinctive habit, attending daily mass, and offering numerous daily prayers, particularly for the souls of the hospitals' founder and benefactors. Those who fell ill or became infirm were looked after by the lay brothers or sisters or servants who did the cooking and washing; in some houses healthy female inmates were expected to help look after those who were unwell. In the smaller leper houses no provision at all was made for looking after the sick.[9]

No medical or nursing care normally was provided at the third category of medieval hospitals either, those that received poor travellers and pilgrims. Knowles and Hadcock listed 136 hospitals (12 per cent of 1,103) of this type, of which about forty-nine probably were intended solely for this purpose and the remainder included poor wayfarers among their inmates. This category of hospital is the one most likely to have been seriously under-enumerated, because many (perhaps most) monasteries maintained a guest house, but only those hospices that enjoyed an autonomous existence were counted by Knowles and Hadcock.

The fourth category of medieval hospital, that intended wholly or partially for the care of the non-leprous sick poor, seems to have been the least numerous. Of the 112 hospitals (10 per cent of 1,103) of this type mentioned by Knowles and Hadcock, fewer than twenty were devoted solely to the care of the sick, and the remainder included the sick among the inmates they received. At least one hospital, that of St John the Baptist, Oxford, also received casualty cases. In 1305 St John's, which was situated near the east gate of Oxford, treated one Robert Attwyndyate, who lived near the south gate, who had broken his finger, and in 1396 one Roger, who had fallen from the nearby East Bridge into the river.[10] A few hospitals, such as St Bartholomew's, Smithfield (London), specifically included maternity patients among those whom they received, and made special provision for them and for their infants; and a few others, most notably St Mary Bethlehem (later known as 'Bedlam'), London, cared for the distraught and insane. One hospital, St Mary Magdalen in Newcastle-upon-Tyne, originally was founded as a leper hospital. According to its chantry certificate of 1546, however, 'syns that kynde of sickness is abated it is used for the comforte and help of the poore folks of the towne that chaunceth to fall syck in tyme of pestilence'.[11] This is the only English hospital that I know of that was intended solely for victims of pestilence.

For most hospitals, however, and in many cases even for those originally founded to receive the sick, the care of the sick became an unwelcome or impossible burden. For example, the statutes of the hospital of St John, Bridgwater, drawn up in 1219 by Bishop Joscelin of Bath and Wells, and exemplified by a successor in 1457, enjoined that the 'poor, infirm, and needy persons in the infirmary' be ministered to by one of the hospital's brothers and cared for day and night by two or three women servants or lay sisters. In this context, however, 'infirm' evidently meant invalid rather than ill, for the statutes went on to stipulate that:

No lepers, lunatics, or persons having the falling sickness or other contagious disease, and no pregnant women, or sucking infants, and no intolerable persons, even though they be poor and infirm, are to be admitted in the house; and if any such be admitted by mistake, they are to be expelled as soon as possible. And when the other poor and infirm persons have recovered they are to be let out *(licentientur)* without delay.[12]

There are many similar cases of the exclusion of both the sick and the infirm. The hospital of St Bartholomew, Gloucester, became impoverished in the mid to late fourteenth century, and by 1381 it sometimes charged for the admittance of the sick.[13] As early as 1316 the infirm brothers, for whose maintenance the hospital of St Bartholomew, Oxford, had been founded, had been supplanted by the healthy.[14] The hospital of St Nicholas, Salisbury, which in the thirteenth century cared for the poor, the sick, travellers, and the infirm, by 1478 had become an almshouse only.[15] Similarly, the hospital at Kingsthorpe by Northampton was founded in 1200 for the reception of the sick and travellers with a staff of a master, two chaplains, and six lay brothers, but in 1535 it supported only two poor brothers.[16]

The hospitals that cared for the non-leprous sick ranged considerably in size and means. The largest was the great hospital of St Leonard, York, whose infirmary was founded to care for 206 sick.[17] It also was the wealthiest English hospital, with an income in 1369 of £1,369 11s. 2¼d.[18] Also among the largest hospitals were the London hospital of St Mary without Bishopsgate, with 180 beds available for the sick at the time of its dissolution; and St Bartholomew's, Gloucester, which in 1333 cared for ninety sick men and women, although by 1535 it housed only thirty-two poor or sick people.[19]

The middle range included the hospital of St Thomas, Southwark, with forty patients recorded in 1295[20] and the same number in 1535; St Mary, Newark (Leicester), founded in 1331 with beds for thirty sick; and St Giles, Beverley, which in 1279 was ordained to have twenty-one beds for the sick, of whom six were to be priests.[21]

Those hospitals that cared for only a few patients included such institutions as Corpus Christi, York, reconstituted in 1478 with seven beds for the sick poor[22]; and St John the Baptist, Winchester, which apparently cared for no more than six sick persons at a time.[23]

Information on admittance procedures for the sick is very scanty. It is recorded, however, that screening of patients did take place at some hospitals. St Mary's, Newark, for example, was founded in 1330–1 by Henry, Earl of Lancaster and Leicester, for five chaplains and fifty poor and infirm folk, of whom twenty were to be perpetual inmates and thirty were to be poor folk suffering from passing ailments and asking the alms of the hospital in charity. These were to be examined at the hospital gate by the warden, who was required to satisfy himself of the seriousness of their complaint and to hear their confession before admitting them.[24] Following a visitation in 1316 of the hospital of St Bartholomew, Smithfield (London), the Bishop of London enjoined the master to order the brothers or sisters of the hospital who were responsible for admitting the infirm to give preference to those who were most in need and not to send them away until they were restored to health.[25] The statutes of the Savoy Hospital in London, founded by Henry VII and completed in or about 1517, required that applicants be screened by four or five members of the staff of the hospital. This screening was to take place each evening for an hour before sunset at the hospital's great gate in the Strand. Of the 100 poor men to be admitted each night the staff were to give preference to sick persons, but they were forbidden to admit lepers.[26] The doggerel poem *The hye way to the Spyttell house*, written about 1536 by Robert Copland, describes the selection process employed by the porter of a London hospital. He attempts to winnow out the genuinely needy – the aged; poor women in childbed; poor men suffering from injuries, the pox, or the pestilence; wayfaring men and maimed soldiers; and 'honest folk fallen in great poverty' – from among the counterfeit lepers and epileptics, the drunkards, the layabouts, the feigned veterans and scholars, the men who pretended to have been shipwrecked, and those who lived from day to day by rotating amongst the various city hospitals. The porter acknowledges, however, that those admitted unavoidably included disreputable men and women.[27]

The names and particulars of hospital patients normally do not survive, except in accounts of miraculous cures, such as those recorded in the foundation book of the priory of St Bartholomew, Smithfield (London), or in those attributed to Thomas Becket.[28] Surviving financial accounts of the small hospital of St John the Baptist at Winchester do, however, record some information about the patients received. In 1351–2, for example, a poor man from Calais lay sick there for fifteen days and died; a poor man was received for thirty-three days, and a poor chaplain for three weeks; six pilgrims stayed in the hospital for four nights; and one Roger Schorham stayed for thirty days. In 1355–6 a poor man lay sick in the hospital for eight days, and a poor boy for four weeks. In 1367–8 the sick patients were listed as three men and three women for seven weeks, three men and two women for four weeks, and so on, for a total of forty-four weeks. Although the system of enumeration used in these accounts obscures the pattern of admission of patients, it appears that from the mid-fourteenth century to the mid-sixteenth century there were no more than six sick patients in the hospital at any one time.[29]

The physical arrangements of the hospitals are better recorded than are their admissions procedures. Most contained or comprised an enclosed precinct, the access to which was controlled by one or more gates. The infirmary usually was built as a long, rectangular hall, like the nave of a church, which it sometimes was called. Usually there was a chapel or chapels at the eastern end of the infirmary hall, so that the patients could witness the daily celebration of mass from their beds. At the hospital of St Mary, Newark (Leicester), for example, the thirty short-term sick inmates were to be cared for in thirty beds lying in the body of the church, from which they would be able to see the elevation of the host and hear the divine offices.[30] The accommodation for a hospital's staff, religious and lay, was separate from that of the sick or other inmates. Almspeople, if resident, might share the infirmary or a common dormitory or dormitories, or might inhabit individual chambers; travellers seem usually to have been lodged with the sick in the infirmary.

Hospitals of this type included St Thomas's, Southwark, references to which of *c.* 1293, 1380, 1387, and 1415 mention the sick and poor lying in the hospital church. In 1400 Henry Yevele, the royal mason and architect, left a bequest to St Thomas's to aid in rebuilding the old aisle 'where the poor patients lie'.[31] The hospital of Kingsthorpe by Northampton had two chapels, with three rows of beds from which poor or sick travellers could hear mass or prayers.[32] Similar arrangements seem to have pertained at the hospitals of St Mary, Chichester; St James, Lewes; and St Nicholas, Salisbury.[33] Ordinarily there was one large infirmary for all patients, although it might be partitioned if patients of both sexes were received. The hospital of St John the Baptist and St John the Evangelist at Sherborne, Dorset, for example, was built by the inhabitants of the town in 1437 with an upper hall for women and a lower hall for men, each communicating with the two-storeyed chapel at the east end.[34] At the hospital of St John the Baptist, Winchester, excavations have revealed a nave-like infirmary partitioned lengthwise into two aisles with a communicating doorway. At the eastern end were two corresponding chapels, which could be viewed by the patients through traceried openings.[35] In some hospitals, such as the hospital of St John, Canterbury, the infirmary hall stood at right-angles to the chapel.[36]

Little is known about the furnishings of hospitals. At the hospital of St John, Winchester, there seem to have been cupboards in the north wall of the northern infirmary that corresponded to the placement of the beds, allowing patients some private storage accommodation.[37] The hospital furnishings mentioned in documentary sources, however, were beds, bedding, hanging lamps, and little else. The infirmary of the hospital of St Mary without Bishopsgate (London), for example, was said to have consisted of a large open ward containing 180 beds, each with its own lamp.[38] An annuity of 5s. was bequeathed *c.* 1293 to the hospital of St Thomas, Southwark, to maintain certain lamps burning in the hospital church before the sick, and in 1415 a Chichester man gave two lanterns to the same hospital to be hung over the beds of the poor.[39] Other bequests were for bedding. In 1540, for example, Hugh Acton, a citizen and merchant tailor of London, left £2 to St Thomas's, Southwark, to buy 'sheets and coverletts for poor people resorting thereto and harbored'.[40] The beds at the London hospital of St Mary Bethlehem ('Bedlam') were supplied with mattresses, sheets, blankets, and coverlets of red and blue worsted.[41] The amenities of Henry VII's Savoy Hospital were unusually handsome. The 100 beds in the hospital dormitory were furnished with flock mattresses and featherbeds, bolsters and pillows; and each had three pairs of sheets, two pairs of blankets, a linen coverlet, and a green and white tapestry counterpane with a red rose in the centre and other decorations. Each bed also had green and white curtains that could be pulled to screen it. The dormitory was lighted all night by three wheel lamps, and earthenware chamberpots were provided for the use of the inmates.[42]

Although one can thus see a hypothetical patient screened, admitted, and bedded down in a lamplit dormitory, near the comforting presence of the chapel, there is very little record of the actual care provided for the sick poor in medieval English hospitals. What does seem clear, however, is that professional medical and surgical practitioners seldom, if ever, treated hospital patients. Vern Bullough found what he believed was an instance in 1340 of a professional practitioner, Master William de Stafford, receiving payments for treating patients at the hospital of St John the Baptist, Oxford. In fact, however, de Stafford was paid for healing the hand of one of the brothers of the hospital.[43] Margaret

Seymour found only two examples of a hospital retaining its own professional practitioners; both were in London, and both date from the sixteenth century. The first of these was Henry VII's Savoy Hospital. The Savoy, founded with great magnificence in emulation of the contemporary Italian hospitals, retained its own physician and surgeon on a part-time basis.[44] The hospital of St Mary Bethlehem, in a letter circulated in 1519 to solicit contributions, claimed that 'the insane, the frenzied and others . . . are lodged and cared for with great diligence and attention, and treated by the physicians with unceasing solicitude'. It is possible that the Bedlam physicians mentioned in 1519 were identical with its masters; three of the hospital's fifteenth-century wardens, John Arundel, William Hobbys, and Thomas Deynman, were royal physicians (Hobbys was also a surgeon).[45]

A physician's or surgeon's mastership of a hospital is, however, no guarantee that he exercised his professional skills on its patients. An interesting demonstration of this is provided by the case of Master Thomas de Goldington, a surgeon who in 1348 held the wardenship of the hospitals of St Nicholas, Carlisle, and St Leonard, Derby. He also exercised the 'office of the surgery of the commonalty', allegedly to the neglect of his duties as warden. A royal commission was appointed to look into the matter, and the commissioners who visited St Nicholas's found that de Goldington was in fact an able and conscientious warden, and that the only defects in his management of the hospital were that he did not reside there continuously, and that there was not the proper number of brothers and sisters. The commissioners also noted that de Goldington 'sometimes exercises the profession of surgery, not to the damage of the hospital, but rather to its profit, because he acquires friends for it'. This suggests that de Goldington took on wealthy private patients, but there is no reference to his treating any of the sick poor in the hospital.[46]

For the period before the sixteenth century I have seen only one reference, again from London, and dating from the fifteenth century, to an explicit provision of professional care for the sick poor. In 1479 the mercer John Don bequeathed the very substantial sum of £25 so that a surgeon, Thomas Thorneton, could continue for the next five years 'in his daily besynes and comfort of the poure, sore and seke pepele lakkyng helpe and money to pay for their lechecraft in London and the subarbes of the same'. This care was to be provided 'in especiall in the hospitalles of Seint Mary, Saint Bartholomew, Saint Thomas, Newgate, Ludgate [both prisons] and in other places, whereas peple shal have nede'. Should Thorneton prove 'slouthfull and nott diligent to attende the pour peple', Don directed that he be replaced by a practitioner willing to observe those conditions.[47]

Outside London I have found no evidence of professional medical or surgical treatment of the sick poor in hospitals. Even St Leonard's, York, with its considerable income and its upwards of 200 sick patients, seems never to have called upon professional practitioners.[48] Similarly, evidence for the purchase by hospitals of medicines or apothecary assistance is virtually nonexistent. The infirmary expenditures of St Leonard's, York, for example, included payments for oil for lamps and lanterns in the infirmary, for candles, and for clothes-washing, but apparently nothing for medicine. The only concrete evidence that Margaret Seymour was able to find that medicine was ever provided for the sick poor comes again from the sixteenth-century royal hospital, the Savoy, the second wealthiest foundation in the country. Among the expenses listed for the poor in the *Valor Ecclesiasticus* return for the Savoy were a number of payments to apothecaries for medicine. The Savoy was the only hospital to list such payments in the *Valor*.[49]

The treatment most likely to have been available to the sick in hospitals was bed rest, warmth, cleanliness, and an adequate diet. It is these provisions that occur time and again in hospital statutes, visitation injunctions, and charitable gifts and bequests. This kind of treatment is exemplified, for example, in the arrangements at Henry VII's Savoy Hospital, where all incoming patients were given a hot bath and a clean suit of clothes to wear while their own clothing was being deloused in two special ovens, and where two fires were provided in the dormitory in winter evenings for the inmates.[50] Ela, countess of Warwick (d. *ante* 1303), left bequests to the hospital of St Mary without Bishopsgate, London, that included perpetual annual payments for the poor in the hospital of £1 for milk, £1 for sheets, and £1 for firewood.[51] In 1458 Stephen Forster, a former mayor of London, left £10, and in 1479 the London mercer John Don bequeathed £13 6s. 8d., to St Mary Bethlehem to be spent on food, drink, linen, and woollen clothing for the sick poor detained there,[52] while two benefactors of the hospital of St Bartholomew, Smithfield, made possible the occasional provision of white bread for the inmates.[53] The foodstuffs purchased in 1363 by the hospital of St Leonard, York, for the poor in the infirmary consisted of wheat, rye, oaten malt, beef, pork, mutton, butter, cheese, and fish.[54]

The actual care of the sick poor in hospitals was the responsibility of the sisters or women servants. At St Thomas's, Southwark, for example, a donation made in 1379 for drink for the paupers and the sick in the hospital was to be distributed by the sisters to whom the care of the sick poor was assigned (*per manus sororum ad custodiam infirmorum pauperum deputarum*).[55] At the hospital of St John the Baptist, Oxford, re-founded in 1234 by Henry III to aid *infirmi* and pilgrims, and 'for the relief of poor scholars and other miserable persons', six sisters were to be maintained to tend the infirm and the paupers of the hospital. The sisters of St John's were replaced in the 1380s, however, by lay servants, two of whom (both women) deposed in 1390 that they served the infirm in the hospital and worked very hard at this (*serviunt infirmis in dicto hospitali existentibus et multum circa eos vigilant et laborant*).[56]

The function of a hospital's brothers, on the other hand, was purely religious. This separation of duties is reflected in the episcopal injunctions sent to the hospital of St Thomas the Martyr, Southwark, following a visitation in 1387. The brothers, for example, were enjoined to conform to the rule of St Augustine, in which they were professed; they were to study the scriptures, the chant, grammar, and the observance of the rule; they were to observe the canonical hours; and, except when saying the divine office or engaged on the business of their house, they were to occupy themselves in the cloister with reading and studying the scriptures. In contrast the sisters, who also were professed in the Augustinian rule, were ordered to supervise the sick paupers daily and visit them personally, which work of piety they were bound to do 'solicitously'. The master of St Thomas's was ordered to check as often as possible on how well the sisters supervised and visited the sick, and how well they ministered to them and fed them.[57]

A few hospitals catered to special classes of patients, and had special facilities for them. The hospitals of St John the Baptist, Bath, and St Michael at Welton, Northumberland, for example, were established for the reception of the sick poor who came to have the benefit of the medicinal waters.[58] At least four hospitals made special provision for maternity patients: the hospital of St John the Evangelist at Blyth in Nottinghamshire, formerly a leper hospital, was re-founded in 1446 for poor strangers and pregnant women[59]; and the three London hospitals of St Thomas, Southwark, St Bartholomew, Smithfield, and St Mary without Bishopsgate also received pregnant women. A taxation survey of St Thomas's carried out in 1295 reported that £1 4s. 0d. a year were spent on coals and fuel for women lying in childbed in the hospital.[60] A fifteenth-century London chronicler mentioned that both St Bartholomew's and St Thomas's had especial care for unwed mothers, and asserted that the wealthy mercer and mayor of London, Richard Whittington, had built an eight-bed chamber at St Thomas's to be used as a maternity ward for unwed mothers, and that everyone in that chamber was strictly enjoined to discretion so as not to hinder the women's chances of marrying.[61] In 1445 the hospital of St Mary without Bishopsgate was described in a papal indulgence as caring for the poor, sick, and miserable in general, and children and pregnant women in particular.[62] A few years earlier, in 1437, St Bartholomew's was given a royal licence to acquire lands and rents in mortmain in consideration of the hospital's 'great charges in receiving the poor, feeble and infirm, keeping women in childbirth until their purification and sometimes feeding their infants until weaned'.[63] In addition, St Bartholomew's tried to rescue babies from the nearby Newgate prison.[64]

Knowles and Hadcock list four other hospitals that cared for special classes of patients. One of these was the hospital of St Leger, Stamford, which was said to have been for the blind, the deaf, the mute, or other infirm.[65] The remaining three hospitals specialized in the care of mentally handicapped, insane, or frenzied patients. These were the hospital of St John the Baptist, Chester, founded in 1232 'for the sustentation of poor and silly persons'[66]; a nameless hospital at Charing Cross, near London, said to have been founded at an unknown date for distraught and lunatic people, whose inmates were unwelcome to the king, who removed them thence to the third hospital, St Mary Bethlehem.[67] Another such hospital evidently was planned for London, for in July 1370 Robert de Denton, a chaplain, obtained a royal licence to found a hospital near the Tower of London for poor priests and other men and women, who had suddenly fallen into a frenzy and lost their memories, until such time as they should recover. Denton changed his mind, however, and in 1378 he obtained another licence to found a perpetual chantry in St Katharine's Hospital instead.[68]

Of these special hospitals, the only one for which detailed information survives is St Mary Bethlehem. In 1403 a royal commission was called to investigate reported abuses there by the porter and acting deputy warden, Peter Taverner. Some eighteen witnesses were examined, including several of the patients, who at that time numbered six insane and three infirm. The commissioners found that Taverner, aided by his wife, had ruthlessly exploited his position in every way possible, and had stolen the entire revenues of the hospital for the preceding four years, and portions of them for the preceding fourteen years. Taverner stole not only money from the almsboxes and food given as charity to the patients, but also everything from bedding to cooking utensils, gardening tools, two keys to the garden gate, a bier, and a complement of four pairs of iron manacles, five other chains of iron, and six iron chains with locks.[69] These presumably had been used as restraints for the patients; an indulgence of 1446 asked for donations to the hospital to support 'the multitude of miserable persons of both sexes dwelling there, who are so alienated in mind and so possessed of unclean spirits that they must be restrained with chains and fetters'.[70]

The kind of corrupt and crippling maladministration revealed by the inquiry into the dealings of Peter Taverner seems to have become a common feature of medieval hospitals, and to have been responsible for the decay and disappearance of many, and the conversion of many more from hospitals offering free care to the sick and needy to fee-demanding almshouses, secular colleges, or schools. Large and wealthy hospitals as well as small and poor ones suffered under this kind of regime. For example, St Leonard's, York, the largest and wealthiest hospital in England, intended in 1364 to care for 206 sick poor in its large dormitory, and to maintain orphans in a hall below, fell victim to the cupidity of its masters, who excluded the poor in favour of those who could pay large sums for places, much of which payments were appropriated by the master.[71] At the large London hospital of St Mary without Bishopsgate, an episcopal visitor found in 1303 that legacies intended for the sick poor were not being paid, that the poor were stinted of their allowances of food and drink, and that the lamps that formerly had hung among the infirm 'for their solace' had been removed. The bishop ordered the hospital to restore the legacies, allowances, and lamps, and added that the lamps were to be provided at the hospital's own charge, and not by selling the clothing of the poor.[72] The hospital of St Thomas the Martyr, Southwark, suffered a number of incompetent and larcenous masters in the fourteenth and fifteenth centuries, culminating in the sixteenth century with the infamous Richard Mabott, a man who abused his position as thoroughly and disastrously as had Bedlam's Peter Taverner.[73] Mabott's contemporary, the master of the leper hospital of St Giles, Norwich, was found in 1541 to have turned that hospital into a sort of Fagin establishment, enticing 'pour lame and diseased personz' into his charge by promising them board and lodging, and then 'when he hath them he compellith them to begge for thir lyuyng or elles they shall have nothing of hym'.[74]

There were genuine exceptions to this very dismal picture. A number of hospitals, of which St Bartholomew, Smithfield, was perhaps the most outstanding, did not succumb to the prevailing pattern of decay and conversion. In general, however, hospitals that cared for the sick poor suffered an extremely high attrition rate, and this process was not effectively counterbalanced in the later medieval period by new foundations or endowments. In fact, the provision of free medical care for the poor evidently was extremely low on the list of charitable priorities in later medieval England. This low priority is reflected in the scarcity of such provision in contemporary bequests, and in the apparent absence of professional care for hospital patients before the sixteenth century, as well as in the falling numbers of the hospitals themselves. Of Knowles and Hadcock's total of 112 hospitals in England and Wales that cared for the sick poor, twenty-four had disappeared altogether by 1535, forty-nine had ceased to provide that kind of care, and in 1535 only thirty-nine hospitals were still providing it.[75]

Notes

1. David Knowles and R. Neville Hadcock, *Medieval Religious Houses, England and Wales*, 2nd edn (Longman, London, 1971) (hereafter K & H), 313–410.

2. Rotha Mary Clay, *The Mediaeval Hospitals of England* (Methuen, London, 1909) xvii, xx.

3. Hampshire Record Office (Winchester), Reg. Stratford, fo. 170.

4. Clay, *Mediaeval Hospitals*, 210; K & H, 325, 334, 335, 371, 396, 398.

5. K & H, 391.

6. Margaret A. Seymour, 'The organisation, personnel and functions of the medieval hospital in the later middle ages', unpublished MA thesis, University of London, 1947, 73.

7. K & H, 391.

8. K & H, 365.

9. Seymour, 'Medieval hospital', 41.

10. H.E. Salter (ed.), *A Cartulary of the Hospital of St. John the Baptist*, vol. 3 (Oxford Historical Society, vol. 69, 1917), xlvi.

11. John Brand, *History and Antiquities . . . of Newcastle upon Tyne*, vol. 1 (London, 1789), 425–7.

12. H.C. Maxwell-Lyte (ed.), *The Register of Thomas Bekynton, Bishop of Bath and Wells 1443–1465* (Somerset Record Society, vol. 49, 1934), p. 289.

13. K & H, 360.

14. *Calendar of Close Rolls, 1313–18*, 323–4.

15. K & H, 389; Seymour, 'Medieval hospital', 60.

16. K & H, 367.

17. K & H, 407; Seymour, 'Medieval hospital', p. 316, citing *Calendar of Inquisitions Miscellaneous, 1348–77*, 202.

18. Seymour, 'Medieval hospital', xxii; *Victoria County History, Yorkshire*, vol. 3, 336–7.

19. K & H, 360, 373.

20. Cecil Deedes (ed.), *Registrum Johannis de Pontissara Episcopi Wintoniensis*, vol. 2, Canterbury and York Society, Canterbury and York Series, vol. 30 (London and Oxford, 1924), 508–9.

21. K & H, 342, 369, 393.

22. K & H, 407.

23. Derek J. Keene, *Winchester Studies. II. Survey of Medieval Winchester*, ii (Oxford University Press, 1985), 815.

24. A.H. Thompson, *History of the Hospital and the New College of St Mary in the Newarke, Leicester* (Leicester Archaeological Society, 1937), 11, 13–19.

25. R.C. Fowler (ed.), *Registrum Radulphi Baldock, Gilberti Segrave,*

Ricardi Newport, et Stephani Gravesend, Episcoporum Londoniensium, Canterbury and York Society, Canterbury and York Series, vol. 7, Diocese of London, vol. 1 (1911), 191.

26. Robert Somerville, *The Savoy* (Savoy, London, 1960), 9, 30.

27. Arthur Valentine Judges (ed.), *The Elizabethan Underworld* (George Routledge & Sons, London, 1930), 1–25.

28. Norman Moore (ed.), *The Book of the Foundation of St. Bartholomew's Church in London* (Early English Text Society, London, original series, vol. 163, 1923), 18, 20, 22–4, 26–30, 35–6, 45–7, 51, 52, 57–60; Frank Barlow, *Thomas Becket* (University of California Press, Berkeley and Los Angeles, California, 1986) 265–7.

29. Keene, *Winchester Studies. II*, ii, 815–16.

30. Thompson, *St Mary in the Newarke*, 13–19.

31. New College, Oxford, New College Archives, MS 3,691, fos 90^r–93^r; John H. Harvey, 'Henry Yevele reconsidered', *The Archaeological Journal*, vol. 108 (1951), 107.

32. K & H, p. 367; Clay, *Mediaeval Hospitals*, 112.

33. Clay, *Mediaeval Hospitals*, 112–13.

34. Walter H. Godfrey, *The English Almshouse* (Faber & Faber, London, 1955), 39–40.

35. Keene, *Winchester Studies. II*, ii, 810–20; Clay, *Mediaeval Hospitals*, 112–14.

36. Godfrey, *English Almshouse*, 33.

37. Pers. comm. Dr Derek Keene.

38. Carole Rawcliffe, 'The hospitals of later medieval London', *Medical History*, vol. 28 (1984), 12.

39. ibid.

40. Hilda J. Hooper, 'Some Surrey wills in the Prerogative Court of Canterbury, 1383–1570', *Surrey Archaeological Collections*, vol. 52 (1952), 37 (calendaring PCC 26 Hankyn, dated 17 June 1534).

41. E.G. O'Donoghue, *The Story of Bethlehem Hospital* (T. Fisher-Unwin, London and Leipsic, 1914), 79.

42. Somerville, *The Savoy*, 31–2.

43. Vern L. Bullough, 'A note on the medical care in medieval English hospitals', *Bulletin of the History of Medicine*, vol. 35 (1961), 76; Salter (ed.), *Cartulary of the Hospital of St. John the Baptist*, vol. 3, 24–5.

44. Seymour, 'Medieval hospital', 48.

45. O'Donoghue, *Bethlehem Hospital*, 100; C.H. Talbot and E.A. Hammond, *The Medical Practitioners in Medieval England, a Biographical Register* (Wellcome Historical Medical Library, London, 1965), 339, 402; A.B. Emden, *Biographical Register of the University of Oxford to A.D. 1500*, vol. 1 (Oxford, 1957), 50.

46. *Calendar of Patent Rolls, 1348–50*, 175–6; *Calendar of Inquisitions Miscellaneous*, vol. 3, no. 6, p. 2; see also vol. 2, no. 1,456, 354–5.

47. Rawcliffe, 'Hospitals', 8 (citing PCC Logge 2).

48. Seymour, 'Medieval hospital', 48.

49. Seymour, 'Medieval hospital', 46–7.

50. Somerville, *The Savoy*, 31.

51. Fowler (ed.), *Reg. Baldock*, 32.

52. Frederic W. Weaver (ed.), *Somerset Medieval Wills 1383–1500* (Somerset Record Society, vol. 16, 1901), 181–2.

53. Nellie J. Kerling (ed.), *The Cartulary of St Bartholomew's Hospital* (St Bartholomew's Hospital, London, 1973), nos. 446, 772 (*c.* 1200 and 1325, respectively).

54. *Calendar of Inquisitions Miscellaneous*, vol. 3, no. 550, 202–4.

55. British Library, Stowe MS 942, fo. 74ʳ (calendared in *Cartulary of the Hospital of St. Thomas the Martyr, Southwark*, Lucy Drucker (trans.) and F.G. Parson (ed.) (privately printed, 1932), no. 231.

56. Salter (ed.), *Cartulary of the Hospital of St. John the Baptist*, vol. 3, xiv, xvi–xvii, xxxi, 7.

57. New College, Oxford, New College Archives, MS 3,691, fos 90ʳ–93ʳ.

58. K & H, 341, 401.

59. K & H, 344.

60. Deedes (ed.), *Reg. Pontissara*, 508–9.

61. James Gairdner (ed.), *The Historical Collections of a Citizen of London in the Fifteenth Century*, Camden new series, vol. 17 (1876), viii–ix.

62. *Calendar of Papal Letters*, vol. 9, 489–90.

63. *Calendar of Patent Rolls, 1436–41*, 48.

64. Nellie J. Kerling, note on Newgate Prison, *Transactions of the London and Middlesex Archaeological Society*, vol. 22, part 1 (1968), 21–2.

65. K & H, 394, citing pers. comm. from Rotha Mary Clay.

66. K & H, 351.

67. K & H, 402.

68. *Calendar of Patent Rolls, 1367–70*, 449; *Calendar of Patent Rolls, 1377–81*, 266; John Stow, *Survey of London* (1603 edn), C.L. Kingsford (ed.) (Oxford University Press, 1908), vol. 1, 137.

69. O'Donoghue, *Bethlehem Hospital*, 76–83; Seymour, 'Medieval hospital', pp. 90, 139–40.

70. Maxwell-Lyte (ed.), *Reg. Bekynton*, 59.

71. Seymour, 'Medieval hospital', 66, 68, 86–7.

72. Fowler (ed.), *Reg. Baldock*, 32–3.

73. Martha Carlin, 'The urban development of Southwark, *c.* 1200 to 1550', unpublished PhD dissertation, University of Toronto, 1983, 405–11; J.S. Brewer, James Gairdner, R.H. Brodie (eds) *Letters and Papers, Foreign and Domestic, of the Reign of Henry VIII, 1536*, 73–4; *1538* (vol. 13, part 1), 494; *1539* (vol. 14, part 2), 301.

74. John Cottingham Tingey (ed.), *The Records of the City of Norwich* vol. 2 (by authority of the Corporation of Norwich, Norwich and London, 1910), 169.

75. These figures are subject to slight revision, because the hospital histories in K & H are abbreviated, and are not always

clear as to the status of individual hospitals at the time of the Dissolution. In some cases, therefore, I have had to make arbitrary decisions in these attributions.

2

Development and change in English hospitals, 1100 – 1500

Miri Rubin

A pioneering scholar in the study of charitable institutions, Paul Bonenfant, expressed his view of the state of research in these words: 'Despite its multiple interests the study of medieval hospitals has not yet given rise to works of general synthesis.'[1] This was in 1965. Two years earlier he had founded the Belgian Society for the Study of the History of Hospitals and had launched its bulletin. Independently and concurrently Michel Mollat of the Sorbonne initiated the Parisian seminar on the History of Poverty, a forum which inspired pioneering works on the concepts, reality, and relief of poverty.[2] These early studies tended to use medieval source material such as theological tracts, literature, civil legislation, canon law, and art, in an attempt to understand medieval poverty. The methodological difficulties inherent in the study of the poor through material emanating primarily from government and from the church soon unfolded, and underlies some of the weaknesses of the early works. An alternative approach emerged in the 1970s, one which used charitable institutions as bridges to the study of poverty. Applied by a number of continental scholars, it focused on asylums, the institutions which harboured, fed, and clothed the needy. These were deemed to be important indicators of some of the options and conditions experienced by the poor. An important attraction was the fact that not only have many charitable institutions left rich archives, cartularies, rentals, and accounts, full of details on every facet of medieval life, but also that institutions of relief, placed as they were at the convergence of religious and social sensibilities of contemporaries, are an important area for a focused yet total view of society. At their best, studies of medieval hospitals can lead us to an improved and indeed new understanding of social commitment, of attitudes towards the poor and towards the clergy, and to an appreciation of the ways in which a resonant message of charity interacted with prevailing and developing economic factors to produce the changing forms of relief. Historians drawn to the study of hospitals, especially in England, could also benefit from a long tradition of local history and of archaeological examination of hospital structures.[3] But there is an urgent need to formulate new concepts and questions and to devise subtle approaches which can do justice both to the complexity of contexts in which hospitals existed and to the diversity of sources relevant to their study.

The rise of interest in hospitals and the poor also coincided with the rise in urban history. The awareness of structural problems of urban life, the peculiarities of its complex social structure, and the importance of towns as venues for experimentation in social and political ideas, as well as in bureaucratic and administrative procedures, underlay an understanding of the ways in which new solutions to old problems were sought. As to the study of poverty and relief, towns possessed a concentration of excess wealth and a close mingling of the haves and have-nots, producing greater need and greater awareness alike. Thus, the urban study suggested itself, with the concentration of institutions and their remaining archives, but, more importantly, as a meaningful conceptual framework for the treatment of what was a network of redistribution determined by a multitude of social, economic, religious, and political circumstances. First among these is Brian Pullan's monumental *Rich and Poor in Renaissance Venice* which demonstrated that the intimate understanding of all aspects of town life – its economy, traditions, social structure, and topography – is vital in any serious attempt to assess its system of relief.[4] Be it a greater commercial centre, a port, an episcopal see, or a university town, its special characteristics affected a town's needs for relief, its ability to give it, as well as the institutional forms in which it could be provided. Thus, studies of poor relief in Lyon, in Narbonne, in Bruges, followed the wake of medieval urban history.[5] And a parallel development occurred in the field of early modern history; we now know much about relief in Lyon,

Aix, Toledo, and Warwick.[6] As urban studies developed a better understanding of the interdependence between town and countryside, and integrated the flow of labour, administrative models, wares, raw materials, ideas, and power between them, into models of urban life, a more complex approach was signalled for the treatment of poverty and relief in towns and their surroundings. Thus, in addition to its local aspects, the study of urban relief should consider several characteristics of the rural neighbourhood; fluctuations in rural prosperity and the charitable solutions which it offered could have immediate bearing on urban needs for relief. The concentration on towns, understandable and necessary as it is, has left the study of non-institutional forms of relief devised by the rural community and enshrined in its customs, awaiting rigorous examination; Richard Smith's interest in life-cycle effects on poverty,[7] as well as Christopher Dyer's contribution to the understanding of medieval nutrition, promise to enlighten us on the structural poverty and morbidity traps which threatened medieval folk.[8]

This paper will trace some of the trends in the foundation and development of charitable institutions in Cambridge and its surroundings. The great wave of hospital foundation in the second half of the twelfth and the early thirteenth century occurred in a period of demographic and economic growth, of urban development, of acceleration of exchange, and the proliferation of markets. All in all it was a period of diversification in economic and social activities. Communal initiatives were taken in new boroughs, in the increasingly effective parish framework, in new village communities, and in old ones where management and exploitation of resources increased in sophistication.[9] These years saw the development of urban institutions promoting and accommodating trade and crafts, and witnessed collective efforts to address their problems of communications, hygiene, and security. In this world of change and prosperity, substantial peasant-holders, manor administrators, master craftsmen, and traders were organizing and improving the environment of their respective towns and villages. Charitable institutions were the result of some of these efforts.

As the community of the borough defined and extended its areas of activity, members explored opportunities in patronage of religious and charitable houses. At least 110 hospitals are known to have been founded in England in towns of differing sizes and characters[10] – in monastic boroughs, in episcopal towns, and in royal boroughs. As the particular, and new, needs and opportunities for urban relief manifested themselves, substantial members of towns and their hinterlands recognized the political advantage, the chance to participate in public activity deemed worthy and rich with social and religious rewards. The earliest attempts at relief looked to existing religious institutions as both recipients and dispensers of charitable funds and as models for organization. Autonomous leper and hospital communities often followed existing guidelines such as parish boundaries, the secular religious framework, or the life of the cloistered religious. The first stage of hospital foundation was a period of experimentation in towns and countryside; and its flexible tentative results provide our earliest examples of charitable institutions.

In Cambridgeshire – and the medieval county boundaries were conveniently almost identical to the diocesan ones – the earliest institutions are two twelfth-century leper-houses, St Mary Magdalene's in Ely and St Mary Magdalene's at Stourbridge, near Cambridge, both mentioned in Pipe Rolls for the 1160s and 1170s as recipients of royal and episcopal alms.[11] The hospital in Cambridge was situated some two miles out of the town centre and boasted a lovely Norman chapel, which is one of the earliest remains of medieval Cambridge. As the need for leper houses probably declined by the mid-thirteenth century, we witness the transformation of these institutions. The hospital at Ely was united to another hospital, St John's, to create a new house living by an Augustinian rule and under episcopal patronage. The leper hospital at Stourbridge had become a free chapel by 1279 and remained in episcopal gift well into the fifteenth century, maintaining no pastoral or charitable duties whatsoever. That England was dotted with such small self-regulating communities of lepers living outside towns, along roads, by streams, and by town-gates, is borne out by stories of houses such as Stourbridge, and by the silent evidence of place names. These typical twelfth-century foundations evolved from a need for segregation tended to by communities of the vills and by burgesses. The treatment of lepers, with its biblical associations, also captured the imagination and largesse of kings and queens, who founded and endowed tens of *leprosaria*.[12] Throughout the thirteenth century, leprosy was in decline and the need for such houses was less pressing: they were then manipulated and transformed by powerful groups and individuals within whose jurisdiction and patronage they fell. In Ely and Cambridge they entered the gift of the Bishop and Priory of Ely. For this the burgess community of Cambridge harboured a grievance and complained bitterly in the Hundred Rolls of 1279; they saw in Stourbridge's demise the loss of an institution which had benefited their town.[13]

The rural institution closest to Cambridge was the hospital at Stow, some 7 miles from Cambridge, founded by the vicar of Stow, and endowed by Sir Aubrey, who appears in the Book of Fee in 1250.[14] This group of maidens, 'the sisters of Stow', wore red habits and possessed a chapel. Similar female communities living outside established religious orders and engaged in charitable works were a common phenomenon in England and the continent in the twelfth and thirteenth centuries. In more formal groupings, layfolk devoted their lives to charity in the third orders related to Franciscan and Dominican friaries. The sisters of Stow are still mentioned in the second half of the thirteenth century and as late as 1338, but seem to have disappeared after the Black Death. This short-lived community was clearly an attempt to provide relief and comfort within the framework of the rural parish.

Another type of charitable provision grafted a group of recipients on to an existing religious house. Some time around 1200 the Gilbertine priory at Fordham was given a messuage, 60 acres of arable and 5 acres of meadow, by a substantial tenant in the parish of Wicken, and in return the house was to keep thirteen poor men in food, clothes, and cover.[15] Such an obligation would have weighed heavily on the purses of small religious houses after a while, and charitable duties were often put aside as memories of patronage and the value of the endowment declined. We encounter numerous papal and episcopal dispensations of the thirteenth and fourteenth centuries freeing religious houses from earlier commitments to relief and hospitality. In some charitable communities the religious element came to dominate and, especially where a rule was observed, there was a good

chance that the hospital would be turned into a full Augustinian priory, as occurred in several places.[16] Charitable experiments were thus conducted in a variety of forms in which
benefactors and founders wished to achieve the greatest possible stability and continuity of endowment, reliable management and maintenance of a religious framework ensuring
perpetual intercession, display, and accumulation of merit.
The instability of many early houses bears witness to the
failure of existing religious houses to provide institutional
forms for charitable foundation which were compatible with
the wish of benefactors for meritorious and perpetual functioning.

With the development of urban institutions, charitable
activity seems to have been naturally drawn into the urban
environment where clearer and more rigorous ideas about
organization of corporate projects, and thus on the management of charitable endowments, were evolving. Thus, in the
second phase of charitable initiatives, in the late thirteenth
century, we witness the rise of a new type of charitable
religious house – an endowed institution which combined the
relief of poverty with a religious and liturgical regime maintained by a regular group of secular clergy and assisted by a
group of lay brethren or sisters. These hospitals were founded
by leading burgesses and supported by a stream of donations
from humbler townsmen and substantial villagers. They were
founded at the entrances to towns, in areas unsuitable for
settlement, on the sidelines of a town's business and social
centre. The permanent community of such a hospital usually
followed a religious rule, maintained a chapel, and soon
needed and procured the ecclesiastical privileges of burial,
bell-ringing, and cure of souls.[17] The evident need for relief,
which was ever growing in the thirteenth century with the
gradual pauperization of a teeming countryside and migra-
tion of workers to towns, was largely answered in such
institutions whose forms were determined by the current
understanding of the organization of religious life. Groups of
canons, or semi-religious layfolk, maintained centres of relief
which offered succour to the poor as well as spiritual benefits
to founders and adherents.

Such foundations were ubiquitous – St John the Baptist,
Oxford, St John's, Bath, St Mark's, Bristol. A leading burgess or group of burgesses would found the house, keeping

its patronage and the right to nominate its master. But the
need for ecclesiastical protection and privilege would soon
turn it into a full religious existence made formal by the
assumption of a rule granted by the diocesan. In Cambridge,
it was one Henry Frost, who by 1204 had given the community of Cambridge what the Hundred Rolls call 'locus pauper-
rimus', a bit of poor waste land beyond the parish of All
Saints, a marshy tract east of the river Cam, which was dried
and filled only decades later to allow the early Cambridge
colleges to be built there.[18] The tradition maintained in the
Hundred Rolls described the subsequent usurpation of
patronage by the Bishop of Ely. Similar complaints about the
loss of control over their hospitals were made in the Hundred
Rolls by the burgesses of Nottingham and Norwich.

Occurring first in 1204, by 1215 the hospital at Cambridge
had become an Augustinian house in the parish of All Saints;
an addition not only to the religious map of thirteenth-
century Cambridge, but also to its business and proprietorial
scene, as an enterprise which people from near and far
wished to join. A period of abundant donation followed the
foundation and the assumption of religious status. Benefactors were not only the leading burgesses but also a multitude
of tradesmen and artisans who gave the new institution
shops, rents, strips in the Cambridge fields, tenements, bits
of gardens, and crofts. They were joined by villagers from the
neighbourhood, the majority of whom resided in villages
within a distance of ten miles from the town, who contributed
acres and half-acres, a piecemeal endowment reflecting the
pattern of their own tenure in the village fields. After a
generation of donation the hospital possessed a considerable
amount of urban property, mainly in the market and in its
own parish of All Saints. Its estate brought the hospital into
contact with other owners, and a sequence of exchanges of
properties allowed it to participate in the active land market
and to consolidate its holdings. In the surrounding villages it
had a fragmented presence, and only in those closest to
Cambridge did it hold more than a scattering of half-acres
and roods. In its dealings and exchange transactions the
hospital aimed at simplification and commutation into annual
rents as far as was possible. Once this was achieved, a striking stability seems to have come over the estate. In the
rentals for the late thirteenth and the fourteenth century most

properties can be traced back to an origin in the first enthusiastic phase of donation in the prosperous years of the early thirteenth century.

The hospital also engaged in a modest moneylending activity. Some loans were forwarded to great men, squire-burgesses, such as the Dunnings of Cambridge, who found that the maintenance of their urban and rural obligations exceeded their income. In such cases the hospital stepped in and provided a breathing space, by freeing them from debts to the Jews and receiving the pledged land thus released as a security. Many such loans turned, in the long run, into donations to the hospital, upon default of payment. When a borrower lost land to his creditor, the hospital, this none the less resulted in procuring the status of benefactor and the spiritual rewards attached to it. Through another instrument the hospital provided credit on a smaller scale; these were in fact mortgages for short terms (between four and six years). Villagers would pledge a few acres, promising to pay a so-called rent for it in a lump sum at the end of the period. The hospital forwarded the sum, usually under 10s. for a number of years, and enjoyed the usufruct during the term of the agreement. These credit agreements were primarily enacted between the hospital and the parishioners of Horningsea, a parish which was appropriated to the hospital at the time of its religious foundation. It is interesting to speculate on the ways in which this lending activity fits into the view of the hospital as a primarily charitable institution. Provision of low-interest loans was often interpreted by contemporaries as an aspect of charitable aid, and the freeing of Christians from Jewish moneylenders was presented in popular preaching as an act of charity and brotherhood. Such activities beyond the purely charitable and religious illustrate the degree to which medieval hospitals responded to the needs of their environment, and in particular to those of existing or potential benefactors.

The foundation and life of hospitals were couched with a terminology and imagery of charity, and those living and working in them were expected to undertake a rigorous religious routine. In the Hospital of St John, Cambridge, a male community was founded following what had become the model of communal charitable life – the hospital statutes based on the Augustinian rule. Augustine's fourth-century set of instructions for communal clerical living was revived in the eleventh century for the reform of clerical living and provided a way of life for a group of priests in proximity to lay society; it was essentially a secular rule, which allowed priests to fulfil functions such as pastoral care, teaching, and charity, and yet to live purely and modestly, to escape temptations, and to observe a full liturgical life. The first to adopt the Augustinian precepts to charitable institutions was the Hospitaller order in the Crusader state.[19] Throughout the twelfth and thirteenth centuries single hospitals took up a modified version which allowed for the coexistence of a religious community with lay inmates and servants, and for flexibility in the routine of those members tending the sick. Hospital rules refer to the life of inmates in varying degrees of detail, and they provide much of our scanty knowledge of the life of the poor and sick. The clauses usually laid down the principles of admission; in the Hospital of St John, Cambridge, these criteria excluded the chronically ill and the permanently maimed: 'We strictly ordain . . . that sick and weak people should be admitted kindly and mercifully, except for pregnant women, lepers, the wounded, cripples and the insane.'[20] Like most hospitals, it assisted the passing sick and poor, those who could benefit and grow stronger and healthier during a limited stay in the hospital, or else die there and be properly buried by the community. Thus, lepers, paralytics, the insane, and those suffering from falling sickness were not admitted, nor were wounded people, and, for other reasons, pregnant women. The rule of the Hospital of St John the Baptist in Oxford explicitly states the rationale behind these stipulations: 'those suffering from falling sickness, ulcers or incurable diseases will not be accepted . . . nor will lewd pregnant women be admitted'.[21]

The incomplete fourteenth-century copy of the rule of the Hospital of St John, Cambridge, does not mention the number of inmates, brethren, or lay brethren.[22] However, the Hospital of St John in Ely, which was given a very similar rule by the same bishop, was a community of thirteen brethren, a master and a mixed lay and clerical community of twelve. In a fourteenth-century list of stipends and later in the clerical poll tax of 1379, both hospitals were said to have a master and five chaplains, which, combined with an equal number of lay brethren, would fit in with an assessment of twelve or thirteen. No surviving material allows us to assess the bed capacity of the Cambridge hospital, but since the inmates were treated in the nave of a chapel divided into four bays, it is reasonable to assume that some eight to ten people were lodged in it, in what is known as the wide-hall form.[23] The rule ordered that inmates be confessed and given communion upon arrival, and like many rules it insisted that they be treated kindly. The strict diet observed by the chaplains, which allowed the eating of meat only twice a week, was to be relaxed in cases where fine and rich meats could fortify the ailing. Unfortunately, only one set of kitchen accounts for the Hospital of St John of Cambridge survives, describing some forty weeks in the year 1343–4; the hospital received grain from its land, and maintained fish-ponds across the Cam, as well as a sheep-fold, but the accounts record regular purchases of butter, eggs, cheese, veal, chickens, and a variety of fish brought up the river. Occasionally purchases of spices are recorded – saffron, pepper, and cumin from the Stourbridge fair.[24]

Gifts to the hospital sometimes stated particular needs: the income from Hugh of Barton's messuage in Newnham was to provide lighting in the inmates' quarters during the night; an episcopal gift granted peat and reeds from the marshes of Ely annually; Harvey Dunning's charter granting arable in Chesterton instructed the hospital to use its income for the maintenance of two sets of bedding. From its fourteenth-century accounts we learn that the hospital employed a cook, a malt-maker, a baker, and a servant. By the fifteenth century a barber, a laundress, and an organ-player were on the payroll. The rule exhorted brethren to keep themselves clean, a clause reminiscent of the rule of St Laurence's, Canterbury, which instructed them to wash their heads at least once a month lest their smell disturb the inmates.[25]

The religious community of the Hospital of St John also maintained liturgical offices and prayers for benefactors, and tended to the pastoral needs of its members and of the parish of Horningsea, of which it was the communal rector. A copy of a fourteenth-century list of benefactors minutely recorded those for whom the brethren were to intercede, a list of names spanning over a century and a half. The hospital was also connected with the Hospital of St John in Ely by a mutual agreement ensuring commemoration for the dead brethren of either community.[26] The non-liturgical nursing duties were filled by lay brethren who were in charge of maintenance, catering, and cleaning, while the more responsible jobs of cellarer and sacrist were filled by the chaplain brothers. The whole community was led by the master, a priest to whom all confessed and all owed strict obedience. Recurrent readings of statutes and weekly chapter gatherings provided the occasion for enforcement of discipline and mutual correction.

The question of medical practices in medieval hospitals is a difficult and puzzling one. One often deals with quite a full hospital archive covering hundreds of years and yet encounters not one mention of purchases of drugs or payments to physicians or surgeons. At the basis of hospital foundation lay the understanding that separation of the sick from everyday life and from neighbours and family was necessary, both for the welfare of the community and to effect their cure. Indeed, the provision of food, cover, a cleaner surrounding, and warmth could go a long way to increase chances of recovery from common illnesses. Little more can be said. In one of the charters of donation to the hospital *c.*1230 one Robertus *medicus* appears as a witness. He may be the same as Robert *le surgien* who held a house in the parish of All Saints near the hospital around 1200. Was he a friend of the donor, or a medical practitioner connected with the hospital? It is impossible to say. In 1279 a university master, Nigel de Thornton, physician, is mentioned as a householder in Cambridge, though he has no explicit connection with the hospital. In 1314 some land in Cambridge was sold to Master Hugo *medicus*; later, in the fifteenth century a doctor of medicine at Peterhouse was paying tithes on his earnings to the parish of Little St Mary. Were these earnings gained from dispensing medical care?[27] The yearly payments of 8s. to a *barbitonsor* in the fifteenth century must be seen as a service to the religious community since by then there were no longer sick folk in the hospital.

The pattern of foundation and development of the Hospital of St John, Cambridge, is characteristic of the initiatives undertaken by burgess communities in the late twelfth and early thirteenth centuries, when urban hospitals were founded in Cambridge, Wisbech, and Ely. It started as a concerted attempt on the part of leading burgesses and substantial landholders to meet problems which were becoming a pronounced aspect of town life such as industrial accidents, sickness among destitute people, and unemployable folk who could not be tended by an extended family or supported by customary mutual help maintained by rural communities. These activities were also couched with religious imagery and promise of salvation, by a spirituality preached and disseminated more frequently and more effectively throughout the thirteenth century. But the efforts for co-operative action and the willingness to apportion a part of one's income and security for the general weal and for spiritual benefits was bound to change once economic fortunes changed and social relations were realigned. By the early or mid fourteenth century the once pauperized countryside was experiencing demographic decline which caused prices to fall, wages to rise, and income from land and trade to fall. The demand for goods and services provided by the towns was slackening, which effected a decrease in the incomes of burgesses. As burgess communities realized that they could no longer easily allocate charitable funds, and that their bounty would be better used in other endeavours, hospitals were left with their declining endowments and, as burgess interest and control waned, with their lax and inefficient administrations. Neither papal directives for reform such as the injunctions published in the collection of canon law, the Clementines, in 1317,[28] nor the episcopal ordinances following visitations, of which there are three sets for the Hospital of St John,[29] could alter the fact that those who had nurtured hospitals were developing different views of their welfare and altered expectations from social and religious action.

The fourteenth century saw the reversal of the process of expansion and population growth and the gradual decline of population by a combination of internal demographic checks, recurrent famines, and finally by the Black Death in mid-century.[30] These changes fundamentally altered the relations between employers and employees, landlords and tenants, and allowed the standard of living of workers to rise while the income of landlords and substantial burgesses was declining. A virulent legislation in an acerbic rhetoric attempted to keep poor labourers in a stable abode and in full employment. In France hospitals came to be used as tools of labour legislation and as locations for punishment and recruitment of able-bodied beggars to work.[31] This interpretation of economic ills as being the outcome of wilful withdrawal of labour by workers inspired a highly suspicious attitude towards all forms of charitable benefaction, which were not closely scrutinized. Thus, hospitals were criticized as assisting the lazy shirkers, and at the same time charitable funds were more discriminately deployed.[32]

In this climate hospitals were obliged to adapt or perish. They were transformed in a variety of ways in order to survive and to suit current patronage choices of potential benefactors. In this process, a burgess foundation of around 1250 such as St John's Hospital, Wisbech, became a royal sinecure by 1352.[33] Many, like St Mary's Bootham, York, turned into chantries for the commemoration of the original founder or of a later re-founder and his family.[34] Some developed educational functions, and many simply disappeared as income from land endowments diminished dramatically in the fourteenth century. Those houses which adapted did so through a total reorganization and redefinition of aims. In the Hospital of St John, Cambridge, inmates are not mentioned after the mid-fourteenth century. The hospital now fulfilled different tasks; its brethren supplied chantry services to burgesses, and served in chantries established in Cambridge parish churches. It continued to provide the cure of souls in the parish of Horningsea, and one of the brethren moved to the rectory permanently. St John's Hospital also accommodated numerous corrodarians, even women, and became the *pied à terre* of the Archdeacon of Ely on his rounds in Cambridge. In 1280 the hospital was the subject of an experiment in academic charity on the part of the Bishop of Ely; Hugh of Balsham installed a group of his favoured students there, only to remove them three years later due to conflict rife between the communities, re-founding the group as the first Cambridge college, Peterhouse. The hospital provided lodging for four university masters during term, and, finally, in 1470 it came to receive full university privileges, allegedly for protection from the harassment of townsmen.[35]

A long road away from the original communal and charitable objectives had been travelled; at its end, and in the particular setting of Cambridge, a group of Augustinian canons observing canonical hours and engaged in commemoration seemed little different from the academic colleges surrounding it. The hospital was assimilated into the liturgical and academic milieu to such a degree that, when it was re-founded as St John's College in 1511, few murmured at what seemed like a natural progression.[36]

While the old institutions, devised in a period of growth and prosperity, combined religion with relief for the poor and sick and were developing away from their original purposes, new foundations were springing up in the late fourteenth and fifteenth centuries which signalled a new understanding of the task and scope of relief. The hospital of Sts Anthony and Eligius of Cambridge was founded in 1361 by the will of a leading burgess and financier Henry Tangmere. His will was to be executed by Corpus Christi College, with which he was associated in his lifetime, and among numerous provisions one was made for the creation of a hospital in two tenements in Trumpington Street.[37] This was to be a leper house, a curious foundation for the fourteenth century when leprosy had all but disappeared, but not one without parallel. The house came to assist all types of disorder, and by the sixteenth century was primarily a small insane asylum. Henry Tangmere's was a lay foundation which did not support a religious community, although it received some episcopal favour in the form of indulgences for its helpers, and had a chapel decorated with paintings and hangings. This clear choice on the part of an astute burgess, to administer his relief programme outside a religious house and without the help of a religious community, falls in with the general trend of distancing from religious houses and employment of the clergy as direct intercessors. The model of St John's Hospital, Cambridge, stood clear before the founder's eyes and could teach a lesson. He chose to entrust the supervision of relief to a perpetual institution such as Corpus Christi, which administered the endowment. Similar appreciation of the power of municipal authorities as brokers in the charitable game is attested by the growing number of charitable and commemoration trusts left to the execution of the Cambridge Town Corporation in the fifteenth century. This movement away from organized religion and towards more discrete and controlled forms of secular relief are expressions of the self-help in religious life, so characteristic of the late middle ages.

A fifteenth-century foundation, the hospital at Newton-in-the-Wash, is yet another form of organization of piety and relief which bore the name *hospitale*. The hospital at Newton was founded in 1403 by Sir John Colvylle as a college of priests and clerics together with some poor men.[38] By 1405 it had received papal protection and in 1411 the parish church of Newton was appropriated to it. In 1452 it was reorganized by the Bishop of Ely, who provided it with a set of statutes; it was to continue as a group of chaplains under a priest as master and to be engaged in the commemoration of the King, the founder, and his family. The master, three chaplains, and four clerks lived in a house attached to the chapel and received generous stipends. The house also accommodated three poor men and a poor woman in charge of all cleaning and cooking for the almsmen.[39] These bedesmen, as the statutes called them, were to live chastely and provide grateful prayers for the founder. They wore habits made of white heavy cloth and were given two pairs of shoes a year. Their weekly stipend of sixpence was paid on Fridays and was supplemented by pittances on feast-days. This house is an extreme example of an institution which offered poor relief as part of a planned and concerted effort to benefit the founder's soul. A lay fraternity was created in connection with the house for those wishing to share the spiritual merit generated by the pious charitable hospital-chantry. No scheme of intercession seemed quite complete, just as no funeral appeared to be well provided, without the presence of the statutory poor, the meek who owed their survival to charitable giving. These poor were not the *raison d'être*; rather they were grafted on to the foundation, and supported by it, just as a single almsman was maintained by the Hospital of St John, Cambridge, throughout the fifteenth century.

Forms of charity and relief were thus re-evaluated and refashioned as the perception of the community's economic well-being and its religious and social aims changed. The shift in attitudes towards poverty in the later middle ages, away from the traditional view of it as virtuous to viewing it as a social menace and a source of disruption, altered the forms in which charity was dispensed. It was no longer through reliance on the good working of religious charitable communities, but rather in more discriminating and controlled frameworks. A multitude of urban almshouses of the late fifteenth century attest to such choices, which were already signalled by a foundation such as Sts Anthony and

Eligius in Cambridge. These almshouses were modest affairs, often located in a house left by the founder, which did not attempt to create a charitable religious unit observing a liturgical routine. It was the bare act of relief, of clearing the streets, of helping the deserving parish poor, that seems to have guided their founders. These almshouses – Daniel's, Lyon's, Jakennet's – offered limited but direct relief, as did their testamentary bequests. In Cambridge, where colleges had emerged as reliable and perpetual corporations, four almshouses were founded between 1463 and 1484; three were supervised by colleges, by King's, Queens', and Gonville and Caius.[40] These foundations survived throughout the sixteenth century and are occasionally mentioned in church-wardens' accounts of the parishes in which they were situated. Such almhouses which carried the names of founders and were managed by layfolk or parish priests under the supervision of executors, guilds, colleges, or town authorities are typical fifteenth-century foundations; they were often conceived as an economic and moral remedy for the homeless poor, for vagrants, migrants, and to the dangers they posed.[41] These almshouses which were founded and controlled by individual layfolk, by gilds, and by town authorities were independent from episcopal supervision and from the intermediation of a religious community. They never developed into the large-scale municipal hospitals and shelters that were maintained by Italian, Flemish, and French towns,[42] but in the English towns they expressed a re-evaluation of charitable aims and means. The choice of the parish framework reflects the preference of an organizational framework based on social ties, co-operation, and responsibility between neighbours; it represented a task of relief which could be controlled and checked by parishioners, family, and friends.

In search of personal and collective gratification and in the attempt to promote the stability and order of their communities, medieval men and women of property and substance allocated excess funds and savings to public charitable institutions. That their willingness to give fluctuated with their prosperity and sense of economic security is abundantly clear. This chapter has shown the resulting changes in the forms assumed by acts of giving and in availability of relief. The study of medieval hospitals and relief agencies has led us on a journey of discovery about the responsiveness of institutions to the values and expectations of those supporting them. It has shown us that a system of relief is little more than the succour which the 'haves' are agreed and willing to provide to the 'have nots'. Institutions relying on co-operation are hit hard when consensus and trust diminish; this was as true in the medieval community as it is in the welfare states of the 1980s.

Notes

1. P. Bonenfant, *Hôpitaux et bienfaisance publiques dans les anciens Pays-Bas des origines à la fin du XVIIIe siècle* (Société Belge d'Histoire des Hôpitaux, Brussels, 1965), 5.

2. M. Mollat (ed.), *Etudes sur l'histoire de la pauvrété*, 2 vols (Publications de la Sorbonne, Paris, 1974).

3. R.M. Clay, *The Medieval Hospitals of England* (Antiquary's Books, London, 1909).

4. B.S. Pullan, *Rich and Poor in Renaissance Venice. The Social Institutions of a Catholic State, to 1620* (Blackwell, Oxford, 1971).

5. N. Gonthier, *Lyon et ses pauvres au moyen-âge (1350-1500)* (Hermes, Lyon, 1978); J. Caille, *Hôpitaux et charité publique à Narbonne au moyen-âge de la fin du XIe siècle à la fin du XVe siècle* (Privat, Toulouse, 1978); G. Maréchal, *De sociale en politieke gebundenheid van het Brugse hospitalwezen in de Middeleeuwen*, Anciens Pays et Assemblés d'états, 73 (UGA, Heule, 1978).

6. J.-P. Gutton, *La société et les pauvres: l'exemple de la généralité de Lyon, 1534-1789*, Bibliothèque de la Faculté des Lettres et Sciences Humaines de Lyon 2 (Les Belles Lettres, Paris, 1971); C.C. Fairchilds, *Poverty and Charity in Aix-en-Provence 1640-1789*, Johns Hopkins University Studies in Historical and Political Science, 94i (Johns Hopkins University Press, Baltimore, 1976); L. Martz, *Poverty and Welfare in Habsburg Spain. The Example of Toledo* (Cambridge University Press, Cambridge, 1983); A.L. Beier, 'The social problems of an Elizabethan country town: Warwick 1580-1590', in P. Clark (ed.), *Country Towns in Pre-Industrial England* (Leicester University Press, Leicester, 1981), 46-85.

7. R. Smith, 'The manor court and the elderly tenant in late medieval England', in Z. Razi and R. Smith (eds), *The Manor Court and Medieval English Society* (Oxford University Press, Oxford, forthcoming, 1990).

8. C. Dyer, 'English diet in the later middle ages', in T.H. Aston, P.R. Coss, C. Dyer, and J. Thirsk (eds), *Social Relations and Ideas: Essays in Honour of R.H. Hilton* (Cambridge University Press, Cambridge, 1983), 191-216.

9. For a study of urbanization in this period see D. Keene (with

A.R. Rumble), *Survey of Medieval Winchester*, Winchester Studies, 2 (2 vols, Clarendon Press, Oxford, 1985).

10. Aggregate figures on hospital foundation are based on the listings in D. Knowles and R.N. Hadcock, *Medieval Religious Houses: England and Wales* (Longman, London, 1971).

11. On the former see M. Rubin, *Charity and Community in Medieval Cambridge*, Cambridge Studies in Medieval Life and Thought, fourth ser., 4 (Cambridge University Press, Cambridge, 1987), 129–35, and the latter, *ibid.*, 111–18.

12. P. Richards, *The Medieval Leper and his Northern Heirs* (D.Brewer and Rowman & Littlefield, Cambridge and Totowa, NJ, 1977).

13. For other instances of patronage losses and disputes see Rubin, *Charity and Community*, 99–103.

14. Op. cit., 135–7.

15. Op. cit. 137.

16. Like Anglesey in Cambridgeshire by 1220, and North Creake in Norfolk by 1208.

17. On the development of pastoral care in the twelfth and thirteenth centuries, see J. Avril, 'La Pastorale des malades et des mourants aux XIIe et XIIIe siècles', in H. Braet and W. Verbeke (eds), *Death in the Middle Ages*, Mediaevalia Lovaniensia, ser. 1, studia 9 (Louvain University Press, Louvain, 1983), 88–106.

18. On hospital locations in general, Rubin, *Charity and Community*, 99–109, 114–16.

19. On the Hospitaller rules see E.J. King, *The Rule, Statutes and Customs of the Hospitallers, 1099–1310* (Methuen, London, 1934); L.Le Grand (ed.), *Statuts d'hôtels-dieu et de léproseries* (L.Le Grand, Paris, 1901).

20. Rubin, *Charity and Community*, 300–1.

21. H.E. Salter (ed.), *A Cartulary of the Hospital of St John the Baptist, Oxford, III*, Oxford Historical Society, 69 (Clarendon Press, Oxford, 1920), 3–5.

22. Printed in Rubin, *Charity and Community*, 300-301.

23. On hospital architecture see D. Leistikow, *Ten Centuries of European Hospital Architecture* (Boehringer, Ingelheim, 1967).

24. Cambridge, St John's College Archive C7.1 (Cartulary of the Hospital of St John), fos 89-90.

25. See the rule of Sr. Laurence's, Cambridge University Library, Add. 6845, fo. 6^v.

26. Rubin, *Charity and Community*, 181.

27. On physicians in medieval English hospitals see R.S. Gottfried, *Doctors and Medicine in Medieval England, 1340–1530* (Princeton University Press, Princeton, NJ, 1986), 259–60.

28. E. Friedberg (ed.), *Corpus iuris canonici*, (B. Tauchnitz, Leipzig, 1879), vol. 2, Constitutiones Clementinae lib. III, 11, cols. 1170–71.

29. Rubin, *Charity and Community*, 171, 190.

30. J. Hatcher, *Plague, Population and the English Economy 1348–1530* (Macmillan, London, 1977), 31–5; E. Miller and J. Hatcher, *Medieval England: Rural Society and Economic Change 1086–1348* (Longman, London, 1978), 53–63; Z. Razi, *Life, Marriage and Death in a Medieval parish. Economy, Society and Demography in Halesowen, 1270–1400* (Cambridge University Press, Cambridge, 1980), 27–32, 114–31.

31. B. Geremek, 'Le Renfermement des pauvres en Italie (XIVe–XVIIe siècle): remarques préliminaires', in *Mélanges en l'honneur de Fernand Braudel. Histoire économique du monde méditeranéen 1450–1650*, II (Privat, Toulouse, 1973), 205–17; idem, 'Criminalité, vagabondage, paupérisme: la marginalité à l'aube des temps modernes', *Revue d'histoire moderne et contemporaine*, vol. 21 (1974), 337–75, esp. 372.

32. On perceptions of poverty in the late fourteenth century see D. Aers, '*Piers Plowman* and problems in the perception of poverty: a culture in transition', *Leeds Studies in English*, new ser., vol. 14 (1983), 5–25.

33. Rubin, *Charity and Community*, 138–9.

34. A.F. Leach (ed.), *Early Yorkshire Schools*, Yorkshire Archaeological Society, record ser. 27 (1898), 33–8.

35. Rubin, *Charity and Community*, 182.

36. E. Miller, *Portrait of a College. A History of the College of St John the Evangelist, Cambridge* (Cambridge University Press, Cambridge, 1961), 1–8.

37. Rubin, *Charity and Community*, 119-22

38. ibid., 142–6.

39. For a similar arrangement at St Katherine's Hospital, Heytesbury, see M. Hicks, 'St Katherine's hospital, Heytesbury: prehistory, foundation, and refoundation 1408–1472', *Wiltshire Archaeological and Natural History Magazine*, vol. 78 (1984), 62–9, 66.

40. Rubin, *Charity and Community*, 127–9.

41. M. McIntosh, *Autonomy and Community: The Royal Manor of Havering 1200–1500*, Cambridge Studies in Medieval Life and Thought, fourth ser., 5 (Cambridge University Press, Cambridge, 1986), 238–9.

42. Pullan, *Rich and Poor*, 202–15; Gonthier, *Lyon et ses pauvres*, 212–23; Bonenfant, *Hôpitaux et bienfaisance publiques*, 39–44.

II

Early Modern

3

The hospitals of late-medieval and Renaissance Florence: a preliminary survey

John Henderson

There have been few comprehensive studies of the hospitals of Italian cities in the later middle ages.[1] This is despite the fact that Italy was one of the few countries in Europe to have experienced a precocious urban development. Cities such as Florence, Venice, Milan, and Genoa, are all supposed to have had populations approaching or in excess of 100,000 before the Black Death, while north of the Alps only Paris was of this size and the large conurbations such as Ghent and Bruges contained no more than 50,000 souls.[2] The relevance to our subject hardly needs pointing out; that it was in these cities that there was the greatest concentration of poor people needing alms, food, and medical treatment. Thus in the later middle ages these centres also saw the growth of poor relief facilities, an important element of which were hospitals.

The term 'hospital' covered a wide variety of institutions, and only some of these were intended to cater exclusively for the sick. The role of late-medieval hospitals should be set squarely within the context of other charitable institutions, including the soup kitchens of monasteries and convents, the social assurance schemes of religious fraternities (either independent or associated with a professional guild), and the more informal systems of parish, neighbourhood, and family.[3] Thus although we shall concentrate on institutions providing medical services, it should not be forgotten that many of the so-called 'hospitals' of medieval Europe were little more than almshouses for the elderly or centres for the reception of travellers and the poor.

Contemporaries and historians have seen the hospitals of Renaissance Florence[4] as in some ways exceptional. The grounds for this are made clear in the prologue to a Florentine law of 1464[5]:

Considering it is said that your city is above all others copiously [provided] with hospitals which are beautiful, and sufficient, and suitable and ordered to receive any sick or well person who is miserable and has need of being given shelter for any reason. . . .

This eulogistic passage was not merely self-conscious humanistic window-dressing. Individual rulers as far apart as Francesco Sforza of Milan in 1456, Henry VII of England in the early sixteenth century, and Emperor Ferdinand in 1546, all looked to Florence when remodelling hospitals.[6] Even Martin Luther, that arch-critic of Roman Catholic institutions, praised Florentine hospitals as 'Regal buildings, with the finest food and drink, attentive service, very learned physicians and clean beds' when he visited the city on his journey to Rome in 1510–11.[7]

If the hospitals of Florence so much impressed the rulers of states in Italy and abroad, was there anything unusual about their evolution or the character of individual institutions? This essay will examine the basis of this reputation. We shall look at the development and functions of hospitals in Florence in the period 1000 to 1500 and also consider the extent to which they may have differed from the hospitals of other Italian states. It will be obvious that we can do little more than scratch the surface of an important subject, which despite the survival of very detailed documentation has, until very recently, remained almost untouched by Florentine historians.

The development of Florence and its hospitals, 1250–1500

An overall picture of the chronological development of Florentine hospitals is provided by Figure 3.1.[8] This is based on a provisional list of either the year of foundation or, when this is not known, the date when a particular institution was first documented.

The dramatic contrast between the period 1000–1200 and the subsequent 300 years may partly reflect lack of surviving

Figure 3.1 Hospitals in Florence, 1000–1500 (by date of foundation or first mention).

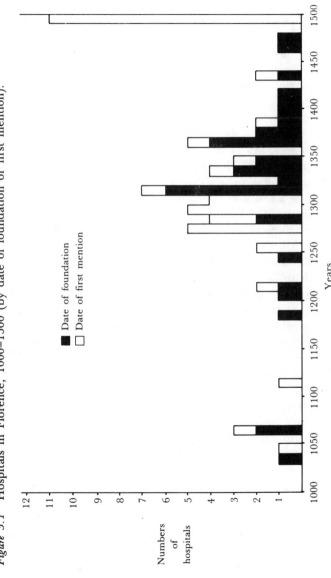

Source: see note 8.

documentation in the earlier period. But this does not mask the considerable increase in the number of new hospitals in Florence between *c*. 1280 and 1350. These foundations coincided with the period of maximum pressure on existing resources. The demographic expansion of the thirteenth century peaked around 1300 and during the succeeding half-century the population of the city was faced with a steady drop in the real value of wages. The foundation of these hospitals reflects one of the ways in which Florentines sought to alleviate worsening conditions among the lower levels of society.[9]

After the Black Death the standard of living improved considerably for the majority of survivors. Florence, like other places, lost at least a third of its population, which fell from about 100,000–120,000 in 1338 to *c*. 70,000 in 1360, and then subsequently dropped to *c*. 37,000–40,000 in the 1420s, as a result of epidemics which occurred at almost ten-year intervals.[10] While lower levels of population may have reduced the scale of poverty, it did not eliminate the poor. As Figure 3.1 shows, other hospitals continued to be founded after the Black Death, partly reflecting the greater availability of cash to finance new institutions.

A graphic presentation of foundations masks a series of important factors, especially the number and size of hospitals in particular periods. A preliminary investigation of contemporary sources reveals that fifty-eight different hospitals were active at some time during the period 1000 to 1500. This does not mean that all these existed at the same time. Like other small associations of laymen, such as religious confraternities, these institutions were often very volatile and may have had rather limited lifespans in the thirteenth and fourteenth centuries.[11]

An idea of how many hospitals were simultaneously in operation can be gained from contemporaries, who also calculated the number of hospitals in their day. The chronicler Giovanni Villani, for example, records the presence of thirty hospitals in Florence in 1338, and the humanist Cristoforo Landini mentions thirty-six in 1480.[12] Fiscal records also give some idea of the number of hospitals in the city, since even exempt institutions had to submit tax returns. Thus the *Catasto* of 1427–8 includes the returns of thirty-five religious corporations termed 'hospital'; the *Decima* of 1495 records thirty-two and the 1527 census of the male population of the city records twenty-nine.[13] It is difficult to judge which figures are more accurate, since chroniclers may have rounded up their calculations, while tax records may have omitted the returns of small institutions. At least it is possible to say that from the early fifteenth century there were at any one time thirty to thirty-five institutions in Florence which called themselves *ospedale*.

This general sketch of the evolution of Florentine hospitals has not yet revealed any feature which makes it markedly different from other cities. The pattern of foundations coincides with that established by studies of other Italian urban and rural areas, and also of other European centres.[14] Nor does the number of hospitals in Florence seem particularly unusual. Florence, like many cities in the fourteenth century, had a ratio of about one hospital for every 1,000 inhabitants.[15]

If Florence was not exceptional in the period of foundation or the number of its hospitals, we should therefore look in more detail at individual institutions to find out whether they had features which differentiated them from hospitals in other cities. This study will be divided into two chronological sections; the first will deal with the period 1000–1348 and the second from 1348 to *c.* 1500.

Hospitals in medieval Florence, 1000–1348

Little detail is recorded about the hospitals founded in the period 1000-1200. A majority of hospitals in this period appears to have been established by churches and monasteries to care for their own personnel, providing infirmaries and sanatoria for sick and elderly monks and nuns.[16] One example was the hospice belonging to the convent of S. Pier Maggiore, which was constructed in 1065 and known as the Spedale de' Pinti. It is typical of the majority of hospices founded before 1300 that we know of its existence through judicial records. The Spedale de' Pinti came to the attention of the court in 1300. The director of the hospice, Giunta Bencivenni, had decided to travel to Rome to attend the Jubilee, and was later discovered to have funded his journey with an unauthorized sale of property, the income of which was intended for the maintenance of the old and sick.[17]

Thus institutions not associated with any offence recorded by the judicial authorities may escape our knowledge.

The largest of these early foundations was the Ospedale di S. Giovanni Battista, which was established in the very centre of the city, between the baptistry and the cathedral, some time before 1040 for pilgrims and the poor.[18] The conditions there in about 1230 were recounted by Boncompagn da Signa, who described the somewhat depressing ambience full of impoverished old men who were given disgusting food and vinegary wine, and were kept awake at night in their foetid beds by the sighs and laments of the sick.[19] Thus although the Ospedale di S. Giovanni Battista, in common with many other institutions of this period, did serve the needs of those suffering from illnesses, this was only one among a number of its functions. It is in this context that one can appreciate the significance of the wording of the statement by the chronicler Giovanni Villani that 'in Florence there are [in 1338] thirty hospitals for the poor and sick'.[20] The poor are placed before the sick in this statement because tending to the sick was seen as only one of the Seven Works of Mercy.

Shelter was the traditional function of a hospital and many of these early foundations provided temporary accommodation for travellers and pilgrims. This is reflected in the location of hospitals throughout the city.[21] In common with the geographical distribution of hospitals studied in places such as Valencia, Arles, Lyon, and Paris, many were founded along the main roads leading into the city.[22] Especially popular locations in Florence included Via S. Gallo, the main entry from the north, and Via Romana and Via S. Pier Gattolino, the two streets leading up to the point of entry for travellers coming from the south.[23] Moreover, virtually all hospitals were established in the suburban area within the city walls constructed between 1284 and 1333.[24] The most obvious reason for this choice of location was that outside the crowded city centre there was space to build. But also of importance was the fact that it was in this area that the poorer inhabitants of the countryside had tended to settle when they came into the city in search of work.[25]

Many of the institutions appearing in Figure 3.1 for the late thirteenth and early fourteenth centuries were founded by small groups of artisans to provide sickness benefit and almshouses for themselves rather than for outsiders. This reflected the policy of most professional guilds and religious confraternities,[26] whose membership among them probably accounted for a majority of the male population above the level of the very poor. Thus in 1317 the porters of Norcia decided to found a fraternity, one of whose aims was to institute a *spedaletto* to be put at 'the service of the poor of Christ', who in practice were their own old and infirm members.[27]

There were two larger hospitals founded in this period which stand out from the mass of smaller institutions – S. Paolo and S. Maria Nuova.[28] The way in which both developed reflects one of the main trends in charity in the first half of the fourteenth century, a movement towards catering for the poor in general. When S. Maria Nuova was founded in 1288 by Folco Portinari there was little to distinguish it from the many other new hospices of the city. The act of foundation stipulated that a house was to be built to give 'hospitality and sustenance to the poor and needy', for whom twelve beds were to be made available.[29] Although treatment of the sick may have been part of Portinari's original aim, the emphasis in practice was to help the poor in general, largely by distributing sums of money to the needy living in their own houses.[30]

Thus by the time of the Black Death, Florence, in common with cities elsewhere, had a series of small institutions which aimed to provide accommodation to travellers and sickness and unemployment benefits to members of those trades and professions represented within the guild structure. Also, like other Italian states, Florence had a number of larger charities which aimed to reach a much wider clientele; the most important were the two hospitals mentioned above and the Fraternity of Orsanmichele.[31] Each one of these institutions expanded its services from the second decade of the fourteenth century, when conditions began to worsen for the poorer members of society.

Hospitals in early Renaissance Florence, 1350–*c*.1500

The demographic and economic crisis of the 1340s has been seen as having a significant effect on charitable institutions in both the short and long term. The immediate effect of the famines and epidemics of the 1340s was a reduction in the scale of poverty. This led to the acceleration of a process which had been begun before the Black Death, a greater specialization in the type of person who was chosen to be subsidized by governments, charitable institutions, and testators.

Even though there were three categories of people who were regarded as equally deserving of charity – orphans, widows, and the sick – there is a common assumption among historians that the Black Death led to the immediate diversion of all charitable funds to medical hospitals. This assumption has to be qualified considerably when one looks more closely at the local level, for the main concern of the governments of a number of Italian cities was the plight of widows and orphans.[32] Many of these people, who had little standing in law, had found themselves in dire financial straits following the Great Plague owing to the death of the main wage-earner of a household and the difficulties in obtaining inheritance. It is significant of the priorities of testators in Florence that the largest charity which distributed alms to the poor in general, the Fraternity of Orsanmichele, should have received bequests worth over ten times the amount left to S. Maria Nuova, the main hospital for the sick – 350,000 florins as opposed to 25,000 florins.[33] It is equally significant that the Florentine government should have passed a law in August 1348 ordering the captains of Orsanmichele to pay the bulk of their alms to widows and orphans.[34]

These two categories of paupers continued to be important recipients of charity in late-medieval and Renaissance Florence. In 1372 the Ospizio of the Orbatello opened with room to accommodate 200 poor women, the foundling hospital of the Innocenti was established in 1419, and then in 1425 the Monte delle Doti was set up to allow fathers to invest a capital sum to provide a dowry for their daughters when they came of age.[35]

Interest in widows and orphans did not preclude interest in the sick, and indeed it has been argued that the Black Death led to an increased 'medicalization' of hospitals.[36] This process can be seen clearly in the case of S. Maria Nuova, the largest and most important medical hospital in Florence. Already by 1348 it had gained the reputation as 'always full of sick men and women, who are cared for and treated with much diligence and abundance of good food and medicines'.[37]

As has been seen, its founder Folco Portinari envisaged its function as providing for all the poor of Christ, but by the late 1320s the hospital was beginning to concentrate on helping the sick.[38] This process was accelerated during the decades following the Black Death, so that by 1374, when the hospital recodified its practices in a new set of statutes, paupers who had no physical disability were not allowed to stay for longer than three days.[39]

The same process can be seen at work in other charitable institutions in Florence. The Ospedale di S. Paolo, for example, gradually moved away from concentration on the poor in general to the sick in particular.[40] Then in the 1380s construction work on two substantial new medical hospitals was begun, S. Matteo in 1385 and that of Messer Bonifazio in 1386.[41]

The period between the Black Death and the third decade of the fifteenth century saw some striking changes in the facilities offered by the hospitals of Florence. Although she shared with other cities the development towards greater specialization of charity, what served to distinguish Florence was the foundation of a series of large hospitals for orphans, widows, and the sick. In order to understand better how these new foundations contributed to the charity available to the poor in this period, we shall turn to their tax returns in 1427–8. Tables 3.1 and 3.2 summarize details about the function and bed capacity of those hospitals represented in the *Catasto*, and include details about other hospitals known to have been active in the early fifteenth century but which cannot be traced in the tax records.

As might be expected, the largest number of hospitals fell into the catch-all category, for the 'poor of Christ'. Three provided beds for between ten and nineteen people, though the majority – for which there is no information – were probably smaller.

The next largest category, hospitals for the sick (21.2 per cent), varied greatly in size, from those with only eight beds to S. Maria Nuova with 230. The smallest was S. Jacopo a S. Eusebio which had been founded in the late twelfth century as a leprosarium.[42] However, with the declining incidence of leprosy, by 1428 this *ospedale* catered only for eight lepers and 100 years later for only two.[43] Most of the earlier large hospitals for the sick were, however, for illness

Table 3.1 Hospitals in early fifteenth-century Florence –
typology

Type	Nos.	%
'Poor of Christ'	8	24.2
Sick	7	21.2
Professional groups	6	18.2
Women	5	15.1
Orphans	3	9.1
Pilgrims	2	6.1
Priests	2	6.1
Total	33	100.0

Table 3.2 Hospitals in early fifteenth-century Florence – number
of beds

Type	Number of beds							
	1–9	10–19	20–29	30–39	40–49	50 +	n/a*	Total
Poor in general	0	3	0	0	0	0	5	8
Sick	1	0	1	2	1	1	1	7
Professional groups	3	3	0	0	0	0	0	6
Women	2	0	0	0	0	1	2	5
Orphans	0	0	0	0	0	3	0	3
Pilgrims	0	1	0	0	0	0	1	2
Priests	0	0	0	0	0	0	2	2
Total	6	7	1	2	1	5	11	33

*n/a = not available
Source: see note 8

in general rather than for a particular disease. This can be
seen from the description of Florentine patients from an early
fourteenth-century sermon by the Dominican Fra Giordano
da Pisa[44]:

> Go also to the hospitals . . . you will see the sick, of
> whom one lacks a nose, another a hand or a foot;
> another who is deaf or blind; another has cancer or a
> fever; while another is in severe pain or is mad; you will
> find a 1,000 miseries and a 1,000 infirmities.

This picture is modified by two recent studies of hospital
patients in Renaissance Florence. These scholars emphasize

that by the sixteenth century these hospitals treated a wide range of diseases, but were designed increasingly for acute illnesses rather than chronic conditions. Of the patients of the Ospedale di S. Paolo, 64 per cent were described as suffering from fevers, and the next largest number (14 per cent) from skin diseases such as scabies.[45]

According to Table 3.1, the third largest group of hospitals in Florence were those run by artisans. The majority were, as has been suggested, on a much smaller scale than both the newer institutions for the sick and the orphanages. Orphanages also tended to cater for a substantial number of children. In 1428 S. Maria della Scala had 151 children in its care, in 1448 S. Gallo had 150, and the Innocenti 700 by 1469.[46] The fifth category of hospital, those for widowed women, were, on the other hand, on a very small scale, with the notable exception of the Orbatello.

Table 3.1 also shows that what are regarded usually as more 'medieval' preoccupations – such as giving shelter to pilgrims – did remain a prominent feature of even later foundations. The Ospedale di S. Lò, for example, was founded in 1435 to provide six beds for pilgrims, each of whom was only allowed to stay for a maximum of three days.[47]

Inevitably categorization of this kind, even if divisions follow contemporary descriptions, are artificial because there was a considerable overlap of function. This can be seen in the 1427 tax return of the small hospice for widows in Piazza di S. Maria del Carmine. Of the seven women present, nearly half were ill and required medical attention. One woman who was aged 80 was described as 'ill and does not leave bed', while another of only 25 was obviously beyond redemption: '[she] has been sick for a year or more and from this illness will not ever recover except when she dies from it (sic)'.[48]

Hospitals in Florence by the mid-fifteenth century were therefore able to provide considerably more accommodation than 100 years earlier. Villani notes that in 1338 there were thirty hospitals with 1,000 beds, which with his population estimate of roughly 90,000 would have provided a bed for every ninety inhabitants.[49] The population of the city probably stood at about 60,000 in the early 1370s, which would have increased the ratio of beds to inhabitants of the city to 60:1. Then by the fifteenth century the facilities for the poor had improved considerably and the per capita:bed ratio would probably have been in the region of 40:1.[50] This was partly because there were fewer people, but also because the city was now served by a series of large hospitals for the sick, orphans, and widows.

It was probably these large charitable institutions rather than the myriad of small hospices which formed the basis for the self-congratulatory statement in 1464 that Florence was a city which was 'above all others copiously [provided] with hospitals, which are beautiful, and sufficient and suitable'.[51] In what follows we shall examine the comments of contemporaries from outside Florence to discover which particular features of the Florentine hospital system they singled out for praise.

The reputation of Florentine hospitals

According to *L'architettura* of the humanist architect Leon Battista Alberti, not only Florence but the whole of Tuscany had the reputation of being 'a land of the oldest tradition of religious piety'. What typified the exercise of this 'religious piety' were the 'splendid houses of treatment built at vast expense'.[52] This suggests that Tuscany's reputation was based on the largest hospitals, which at the time he was writing in the 1440s meant S. Maria Nuova in Florence and S. Maria della Scala in Siena.[53] Other contemporary evidence confirms this assumption. For example, a Bull of 1449 gave the confraternity of S. Matteo in Pavia papal approval to erect a hospital in the city which was to be designed 'with a chapel, bells and cemetery for the poor . . . in the likeness of the hospitals of Florence and Siena'.[54]

Again in 1456, during the planning of the Ospedale Maggiore in Milan, the Duke, Francesco Sforza, asked his ambassadors for details of the hospitals of Siena and Florence.[55] He was clearly interested in every aspect of their organization and appearance. The report of the Sienese ambassador included details of the personnel, the income, and the layout of S. Maria della Scala.[56] Sforza then wrote to Giovanni de' Medici in Florence to explain that because 'in this our city of Milan a large hospital has been begun' he was sending to Florence the architect of the

Ospedale Maggiore, Filarete, together with Giovanni di Sant'Ambrogio, 'so that they might see in its entirety all that hospital of that your city [presumably S. Maria Nuova], and in order to examine it and to obtain [a copy of] the design'.[57] In this way it was hoped 'we may produce the best design that will be possible'.[58]

There appear to be conflicting views among architectural historians concerning the exact nature of the influence of these two great Tuscan hospitals. Traditionally it has been assumed that S. Maria Nuova's cruciform groundplan inspired Filarete's design of the Ospedale Maggiore in Milan.[59] However, it has been pointed out that S. Maria Nuova did not have a completed cruciform groundplan for twenty-three years after the planning of the Ospedale Maggiore.[60] Even so, the two Tuscan hospitals may have been more influential than this suggests. First, the design of S. Maria Nuova, which was so carefully inspected by Filarete, probably already included a plan to extend the existing structure – an inverted L-shape – to form a cross.[61] Secondly, the 1456 description of S. Maria della Scala indicates that it definitely did have two wards connected by a corridor to form the shape of a cross.[62] These two hospitals were, however, not the most immediately obvious models for the Ospedale Maggiore; by 1456 there were two cruciform hospitals being built much closer than Florence, in Pavia and Mantua.[63] At the present state of research, however, it is difficult to make a definitive statement about the possible influence of any Tuscan cruciform designs on the hospitals of northern Italy.

Hospital designers of northern Italy of the mid-fifteenth century evidently did see themselves as indebted to the models provided by Tuscany. It was above all the scale of these institutions which impressed them. S. Maria Nuova and S. Maria della Scala were dominated by two long wards for the male and female patients respectively. By the middle of the fifteenth century S. Maria della Scala catered in just one of these *corsie* for 130 male patients and pilgrims, and S. Maria Nuova treated each month more than 300 patients.[64] Further important parts of these large hospital complexes included service areas such as the kitchens, laundries, and pharmacies, and accommodation for the resident staff, many of whom were members of a religious order.

Finally another characteristic of Florentine hospitals which was imitated elsewhere was their porticoed facades. The most well-known example was that of the Ospedale degli Innocenti, where the *loggia* acted as the intermediary space between the public street and the private world of the residents.[65]

However innovative the scale and design of these new Renaissance hospitals, it should not be forgotten that all were based on a medieval ecclesiastical model. The wards were based on the plan of a church, emphasized by placing an altar at the head of the nave or, in the case of a cruciform design, at the meeting-point of the four arms of the cross. This was to have both a practical and spiritual purpose, in order that the medical staff could have a clear view of all the patients and that the latter could always be able to see Mass being celebrated. The ecclesiastical model was further emphasized by the invariable inclusion of a cloister, which often separated the two main wards and was designed for the use of the members of the order who ran the hospital.[66]

But it was not just the design of the hospitals which interested people from outside Tuscany. Both the report on S. Maria della Scala for Francesco Sforza and the copy of the ordinances of S. Maria Nuova prepared for Henry VII of England include detailed information about administration and finance.[67] These two subjects will form the basis of the final section.

The finance and administration of Florentine hospitals

The finances of many religious corporations in early fifteenth-century Florence appear in their tax returns of 1427–8. Even though exempt as a 'luogo pio', each hospital had to submit a detailed account of all its assets and main financial obligations. Using these returns to assess the relative wealth of hospitals in Pistoia, one historian concluded that they were by far the richest corporations in the city. The budget of the large Ospedale del Ceppo, for example, was nearly twice that of the very considerable budget of the Bishop.[68] The same is true of Florence. Although the complete *Catasto* return for the city's largest hospital, S. Maria Nuova, does not survive, a century later it was estimated that its annual income from its possessions was 25,000 florins.[69] Even if its income had been only half as large in 1428, its capital would still have amounted to 178,571 florins or five times the total capital of the largest ecclesiastical entity in the city, the archbishopric and cathedral canons.[70]

Although the capital of other Florentine hospitals did not approach that of S. Maria Nuova, both S. Gallo and S. Bonifazio, at 13,557 and 15,527 florins respectively, held substantial assets.[71] It is instructive that this placed these hospitals at about the same level of wealth as the largest charitable confraternity of the city, Orsanmichele with 14,947 florins, and not much less than the combined assets of the two companies of the Misericordia and Bigallo with 18,085 florins.[72] Another of the new hospitals, that of S. Matteo, had capital worth 8,186 florins, only just lower than the largest and most affluent canonical church, S. Lorenzo (9,359 florins), patronized heavily by the Medici family.[73] However, as with most Florentine parishes and confraternities, many of the city's hospitals had assets valued at well below 300 florins. These ranged from the Ospedale di SS. Jacopo e Filippo in Via Porcellana with assets of 249 florins and S. Salvadore with 225 florins, down to S. Lucia with only 64 florins.[74]

The main assets of most hospitals consisted of property in the city and countryside, although the larger institutions tended to diversify their financial investments. Property consisted of private houses, commercial shops and stalls in the marketplace, and farms, fields, and vineyards in the Florentine *contado*.[75] The more enterprising directors of the larger hospitals managed their assets with a view to maximizing their output. Research on the records of the orphanage of S. Gallo, for example, reveals a deliberate policy of rationalizing landholdings over a number of years, mostly by selling off far-flung parcels of land and buying up farms in an area just north of the city. In this way the land could be farmed more efficiently and fresh produce for patients procured at a shorter distance.[76]

Larger institutions, such as S. Maria Nuova, also became involved in a whole series of investment strategies, partly through inheritance and partly through deliberate policies of individual directors. Hospitals, in common with large charities such as Orsanmichele, were left not just property, but also shares in the *Monte Comune* or the city's communal debt.[77] And from 1464 S. Maria Nuova itself offered a service to investors; interest of 5 per cent was paid to anybody who deposited money with the hospital.[78] Evidently the handling of such large sums could lead to abuses, for in 1527 the director of S. Maria Nuova was dismissed for allowing his Medicean friends access to the funds which they then proceeded to lend to the commune for a return of 14 per cent.[79]

Although the contemporary chronicler, Giovanni Cambi, remarked dismissively of this affair 'and this was the charity and love they bore their country',[80] hospitals did not view financial dealings as inconsistent with charity, and often combined them. Most important were the retirement contracts it offered to the elderly. Frequently widows, short of cash to meet their everyday living expenses, made over their property to a hospital in return for a guaranteed income for the rest of their lives.[81]

Although the surviving financial records of a hospital such as the Ceppo or S. Maria Nuova suggest that large sums passed through their treasurers' hands, this does not necessarily mean that the hospital itself was thereby enriched.[82] As in the case of S. Maria della Scala in Siena, it was quite possible for an institution to be appointed as executor of substantial legacies, the proceeds of which then had to be distributed to the relatives of the deceased or even to other pious institutions. In this way little might be left for the executing institution, the hospital, or religious confraternity.[83] This becomes clear when examining the expenses and obligations of hospitals represented in the *Catasto*, as can be seen in the case of the Ospedale di S. Matteo (see Table 3.3).

S. Matteo was very much in debt, which is somewhat surprising considering that it had been founded only forty-two years before. Although it had substantial holdings – twelve houses of various sizes, nineteen farms, four vineyards, and three shops – a large number of people owed money to it. At the end of its tax return was written 'From all the above listed debtors it is impossible to collect one penny either because he is dead or has gone away or has gone bankrupt . . . so we have to conclude that these debts are lost.'[84] While it would be easy to conclude from this lament that the hospital was exaggerating the parlous state of its finances in order to protect itself against the depredations of

Table 3.3 Income and expenditure of the Ospedale di S. Matteo
in 1428 (all amounts are in florins)

	Amount	%
Income		
Total annual income	573	100
Expenditure		
1. *Salaries*		
4 priests	41	2.8
2 doctors	15	1.0
1 factor	24	1.6
	80	5.4
2. *Expenses for attendants and servants*		
Food	432	29.5
Clothes	125	8.5
	557	38.1
3. *Expenses for patients*		
Food at 15 florins p.a. for 45 patients	675	46.2
Bed repairs and medicine	70	4.8
	745	51.0
4. *Maintenance*		
Building repairs	40	2.7
Repairs to household objects	10	0.7
	50	3.4
5. *Church services*	11	0.8
6. *Legatees*	19	1.3
Total annual expenditure	1,462	100.0
Balance	− 889	

Source: Catasto 185.2, ff. 601^r, 607^r; see note 8

future tax officials, this picture is confirmed by the returns of
other hospitals. The Ceppo in Pistoia, for example, had a
deficit of roughly 525 florins, the Innocenti complained that
it had incurred a debt of more than 100 florins because of the
expenses of building, and the Spedale de' Preti told the tax
officials 'Do not marvel' that expenditure on its hospital
exceeded its income.[85]
    S. Matteo's largest single item of expenditure was the
maintenance of the patients, although food (at 46.2 per cent
of total expenditure) far exceeded medicine (at 4.8 per cent,
which included repairs to beds). While the daily fare listed in
these hospitals account books does not seem very different

from that of a typical trattoria today, it was a considerable improvement over the diet of the average Florentine; it included meat, poultry, fish, grain, fresh fruit, and vegetables, as well as a substantial amount of wine.[86] It is usually difficult to distinguish the food provided for employees from that for patients, but the records of S. Maria Nuova suggest that a major medical hospital tended to feed its patients mainly on a diet in which chicken broth and eggs predominated; in the early sixteenth century the hospital purchased each year 40,000 chickens and 80,000 eggs.[87]

The rest of the expenditure was concerned with running the hospital, an important part of which was paying salaries and the maintenance of the live-in staff. Information from the *Catasto* concerning the hospital personnel reveals a similar administrative structure for all Florentine hospitals. Each was headed by a *spedalingo* or director. He was helped by assistants, varying in number according to the size of the institution; these included staff to help with the administration of the hospital, as well as clergy to perform the holy office, gardeners to till the soil, and a medical staff of doctors and nurses to tend to the inmates.[88]

The *spedalingo* established the reputation of a hospital and dictated its fortunes. Most remain fairly shadowy figures, but some particularly active *spedalinghi* do stand out. Two especially well-known figures of the late fifteenth and early sixteenth centuries are the priest Benino de' Benini and Lionardo Buonafe, a monk and later Bishop of Cortona. Benini has emerged from a recent study of S. Paolo as the driving force behind the development of the hospital and the redesign of the whole building complex, while Buonafe has traditionally been portrayed as the man who restored the flagging finances of S. Maria Nuova, increased considerably its revenues, and extended the facilities available for the sick.[89] One characteristic both men shared with the directors of the smaller hospitals was that they stayed in office until they were elderly. The average age of the *spedalinghi* of seven smaller Florentine hospices was 65, with two of them over 80; each was a layman who was married to a woman on average eight years his junior.[90] It may well be that these posts were seen as most suitable for the retired, a way of providing free board and lodging for one more elderly couple.

Just as hospital directors were professional religious or

laymen without any medical training, so were the nursing staff. This is not surprising, given that looking after the sick was seen in this period as only one of an number of ways in which a layman could help the poor. Their role was to 'give shelter . . . to the sick poor who come to the hospital, as they would to Christ himself'.[91] The main qualification for those who chose to work full-time as nurses in a hospital was therefore complete dedication. Many of the nurses at the larger hospitals lived on the premises and were members of a religious order, such as the Franciscan Tertiaries of S. Paolo or the male *conversi* and female oblates of S. Maria Nuova.[92]

Many of the larger Florentine hospitals seem to have had a substantial number of live-in nurses: Messer Bonifazio had a patient population of thirty-one who were tended by six male and twenty female nurses; S. Matteo's forty-five patients were looked after by thirty-six men and women; and S. Maria Nuova, without counting male staff and with a bed capacity of 230, had 100 female nurses.[93] While this ratio may seem high even by modern standards, one should not forget that hospitals were also providing a charitable service to those whom they employed. Single women, and in particular widows, found themselves frequently on a very low income; the fact that they received free board and lodging may have been as great an incentive to dedicate themselves to serve the sick poor as the possibility that later they too might receive support in old age.

In addition to nurses, medical staff included doctors; indeed, their presence in a hospital can be taken to distinguish them as institutions which treated the sick from the more general almshouses. Most doctors appear to have been paid on a retainer and therefore received low salaries. For example, S. Maria della Scala paid its Maestro Benedetto *medicho* 16 bushels of wheat, which was equivalent to about 3 florins, while the hospital's barber-surgeon, Antonio di Giuliano, received 2.5 florins.[94] These sums would have represented probably no more than 3 per cent of the annual income of what has been described as a 'medium level physician',[95] which also suggests that many doctors may have charged less for their professional services, seeing their work in hospitals as an act of charity.

One hundred years later doctors in S. Maria Nuova received higher salaries; physicians were paid 24 florins a year and barber-surgeons 14 florins.[96] Judging from the hospital's early sixteenth-century ordinances, this was partly because the large number of patients made these doctors' duties more onerous, and partly because they were chosen from among the six 'most excellent in all the city'.[97] These men visited the hospital on a daily basis and prescribed the relevant treatment and medication, which was then administered by the nurses and supervised by three junior doctors, who provided their services free of charge in exchange for board and lodging and the opportunity to gain direct clinical experience. Finally, a surgeon came daily to the hospital to treat 'those with sores [i.e. skin lesions]' and the wounded.[98]

As in most large hospitals, female patients were housed in a separate ward and looked after by women rather than men. In addition to nurses, a female 'magistra' was employed who 'has experience in these things', as well as a woman who was 'well skilled in surgery'.[99] Little is known about these medical women, although it is possible that they had gained experience through living in the hospital and in this way, as the compiler of the ordinances somewhat incredulously remarks, they achieved 'many cures [which] are remarkable and indeed incredible'.[100]

Towards a conclusion

It is hard not to come away from examining the ordinances of S. Maria Nuova without an optimistic view of patient care in Renaissance Florence. This picture would seem to be confirmed by recent studies of the Ospedale di S. Paolo and S. Maria Nuova, which show that patients stayed on average only eleven to fifteen days and that 80 to 90 per cent were cured and returned home.[101] Furthermore, the overall picture which has emerged from this brief survey of the various stages in the development of Florentine hospitals points to the gradual improvement and expansion in the facilities available to the poor and sick. In particular, after the mid-fourteenth century, with the reduction in the scale of poverty, there was an increased opportunity for greater specialization in the distribution of poor relief. Charitable institutions, including fraternities and hospitals, began to concentrate on helping not just the traditional biblical categories of orphans and widows, but also the sick. In addition to the expansion of existing hospitals, new ones emerged which impressed contemporaries by the scale of their operation and design. It was these large hospitals which formed the basis of Florence's reputation abroad.

However, it must be borne in mind that many of the sources which have so far been used by historians when assessing the services provided by Florentine hospitals tend to have been literary or even oratorical in origin.[102] They include comments by chroniclers like Villani, or by a chancellor of the Florentine state like Leonardo Bruni,[103] or humanists such as Alberti or Landini. Other sources are more overtly propagandist in intention, such as the prologues of contemporary laws. Even Luther's eulogistic description of the treatment he is presumed to have received in S. Maria Nuova would hardly have been representative of the experience of the patients of all Florentine hospitals. The features he described included the 'finest food and drink', 'beautifully painted beds', and 'gentlewomen in veils' who nursed the patients. But it is possible that these services may have been only available to the inmates of the *Sapientia*, the room especially reserved for the clergy, rather than to the average sick pauper.[104] Indeed when discussing the ordinances of S. Maria Nuova, one should not forget that they were probably prepared to impress a foreign monarch, Henry VII of England.

This study has also shown that other types of documents can reveal rather different and less optimistic aspects of the same picture. The *Catasto* returns of, for example, even a relatively new hospital such as S. Matteo show a charitable institution struggling to meet mounting debts. Further work on the very rich financial records of other hospitals may well indicate more widespread indebtedness than we are aware of at the present state of research. These institutions, which often relied for the bulk of their income on fixed assets, could easily go through periods of decline, especially as a result of maladministration or the inability to collect rent. Thus in 1444 a letter from the Florentine government stated that the finances of some of the main hospitals of the city were strained: 'because of the quantity of miserable people, and the [abandoned] male and female children to feed, they [the hospitals] are only able to meet their needs and necessities with the greatest difficulty'.[105]

83

Their resources were stretched even further during famines and epidemics. During the 150 years following the Black Death, epidemics recurred at almost ten-year intervals.[106] On each of these occasions existing hospitals bore the initial brunt of the problems caused by the sudden proliferation of sick people.[107] Although governments provided subsidies for hospitals, their facilities proved very inadequate and by 1464 the Florentine regime recognized that by placing plague victims in S. Maria Nuova 'it harms the others who are sick from another infirmity'.[108] However, when the much trumpeted solution of building a separate *Lazzaretto* for plague victims was finally realized some time after 1479, its capacity was so minimal that existing charitable institutions continued to be the principal agencies to cater for the sick during epidemics.[109]

The lack of a *Lazzaretto* in 1464 was regarded at that time as the major flaw in the facilities offered by hospitals in Florence. But while their hospitals continued to be admired as 'more beautiful and sufficient and suitable' than those of other cities,[110] by the second half of the fifteenth century many Italian city-states were founding their own large institutions which could rival the facilities available in Florence. The famous cruciform design soon became a standard feature of many institutions in northern Italy and it was the Ospedale Maggiore of Milan rather than S. Maria Nuova or S. Maria della Scala which architectural historians see as being 'among the six most influential hospital designs in the world'.[111] Moreover elsewhere, and particularly in Lombardy, there was a move towards rethinking the way in which hospitals were organized. Instead of the myriad of small institutions so familiar to many late-medieval towns, city-states began to establish more centralized systems by uniting the smaller hospitals into a coherent framework controlled from the centre.[112] However, despite Tuscany's reputation for charity, it was not until the middle of the sixteenth century that the grand-dukes began to follow the lead of other states and centralize their poor-relief facilities.[113] Whether this really did lead to an improvement in the facilities available to the poor and sick must remain open to debate when the basic research on so many aspects of the history of Florentine hospitals still needs to be completed.

Notes

1. I am grateful to Richard Goldthwaite, Katharine Park, and Patrick Sweeney for their comments on an earlier version of this paper, which was written while the author was a Wellcome Trust Fellow at the Wellcome Unit for the History of Medicine, University of Cambridge.

All manuscripts, unless otherwise stated, are in the Archivio di Stato di Firenze.

Until very recently the best studies of hospitals in southern Europe have tended to have been sections of books on wider issues, such as: B. Pullan, *Rich and Poor in Renaissance Venice. The Social Institutions of a Catholic State to 1620* (Oxford, 1971); I. Naso, *Medici e strutture sanitarie nella società tardo-medievale. Il Piemonte dei secoli XIV e XV* (Milan, 1982); L. Martz, *Poverty and Welfare in Habsburg Spain. The Example of Toledo* (Cambridge, 1983). For Spain see now: D. Jetter, *Spanien von den Anfangen bis um 1500. Geschichte des Hospitals*, IV (Stuttgart, 1980); and *Drei spanische Kreuzhallenspitäler und Ihr Nachhall in aller Welt* (Stuttgart, 1987). See also U. Lindgren, *Bedürftigkeit, Armut, Not: Studien zur Spätmittelalterlichen sozialgeschichte Barcelonas* (Munster, 1980); and A. Rubio Vela, *Pobreza, enfermedad y asistencia hospitaria en la Valencia del siglo XIV* (Valencia, 1984).

Although in the past most studies of Italian hospitals have been merely descriptive, recently more analytical monographs of individual hospitals have begun to appear, based on careful archival research. For example: L. Grassi, *Lo 'spedale di poveri' del Filarete* (Milan, 1972); M.O. Banzola, *L'ospedale vecchio di Parma* (Parma, 1980); *Lo spedale Serristori di Figline. Documenti e arredi* (Figline, 1982); S. Lunerdon (ed.), *Hospitale S. Marie Cruciferorum. L'ospizio dei crociferi a Venezia* (Venice, 1985); L. Sandri, *L'Ospedale di S. Maria della Scala di S. Gimignano nel Quattrocento. Contributo alla storia dell'infanzia abbandonata* (Florence, 1982); S.R. Epstein, *Alle origini della fattoria toscana. L'ospedale della Scala di Siena e le sue terre (metà '200- metà '400)* (Florence, 1986); M. Heinz, 'San Giacomo in Augusta in Rom und der Hospitalbau der Renaissance' (PhD diss., Rheinischen Friedrich-Wilhelms-Universität zu Bonn, 1977).

2. N.J.G. Pounds, *An Economic History of Medieval Europe* (London, 1974), 258–9.

3. For a valuable general introduction to charity in Italy see B. Pullan, 'Poveri, mendicanti e vagabondi (secoli XIV–XVII)', *Storia d'Italia. Annali 1. Dal feudalesimo al capitalismo.* (Turin, 1978), 981–1,047. See also the following collections of essays on the subject: T. Riis (ed.), *Aspects of Poverty in Early Modern Europe* (Stuttgart, 1981); G. Politi, M. Rosa, F. della Peruta (eds) *Timore e carità. I poveri nell'Italia moderna* (Cremona, 1982); and 'Charity and the poor in Medieval and Renaissance Europe', in J. Henderson (ed.), *Continuity and Change*, 3 (2) (1988).

4. The only comprehensive survey of hospitals in Florence is still L. Passerini, *Storia degli stabilmenti di beneficenza e d'istruzione elementare gratuita della città di Firenze* (Florence, 1853). A few useful studies have appeared recently of individual hospitals: the general book by G. Pampaloni, *Lo spedale di Santa Maria Nuova* (Florence, 1961); R.A. Goldthwaite and W.R. Rearick, 'Michelozzo and the Ospedale di San Paolo in Florence', *Mitteilungen des Kunsthistorischen Institutes in Florenz*, XXI (1977), 221–306; R.C. Trexler, 'Infanticide in Florence: new sources and first results', *History of Childhood Quarterly. The Journal of Psychohistory*, 1 (1973–74), 96–116, and 'The foundlings of Florence, 1395–1455', op. cit., 259–84; B.J. Trexler, 'Hospital patients in Florence: San Paolo, 1567–68', *Bulletin of the History of Medicine*, XLVIII (1974), 41–59. Other recent works tend to be of short descriptive articles: M.A. Mannelli, 'Istituzione e soppressione degli ospedali minori in Firenze', *Ospedali d'Italia. Chirurgia*, 12 (1965), *Studi di storia ospitaliera*, 111 (1965), 171–82; Mannelli, 'L'Ospedale di Sant'Antonio in Firenze', 505–8; Mannelli, 'Lo spedale di San Paolo dei convalescenti in Firenze, *Ospedali d'Italia. Chirurgia*, 12 (1965), 241–5; E. Coturri, 'L'Ospedale così detto ''di Bonifazio'' in Firenze', *Pagine di storia della medicina*, 3 (1959), 15–33; Mannelli, 'L'ospedale di San Matteo in Firenze', *Ospedali d'Italia. Chirurgia*, 11 (1964), 730–2.

5. A. Corsini, *La morìa del 1464 in Toscana e l'institutione dei primi lazzaretti in Firenze ed in Pisa* (Florence, 1911), 34: 12 June 1464.

6. P. Foster, 'Per il disegno dell'Ospedale di Milano', *Arte Lombarda*, 38–9 (1973), 9–10; Passerini, pp. 851, 867. Passerini mistakenly suggests that the description of S. Maria Nuova was prepared for Henry VIII.

7. Quoted in R. Friedenthal, *Luther* (London, 1967), 78.

8. The sources consulted to compile Figure 3.1 and Tables 3.1, 3.2 and 3.3 are partly published and partly unpublished. See the references in R. Davidsohn, *Storia di Firenze*, trans. G.B. Klein (Florence, 1972), VII, 87–104 and G. Fanelli, *Firenze, architettura e città. Atlante* (Florence, 1973), 154: Passerini, *Storia*; W. and E. Paatz, *Die Kirchen von Florenz* (Frankfurt-am-Main, 1954), 6 vols; and M. Giusti and P. Guidi (eds), *Rationes decimarum Italiae: Tuscia. Le decime degli anni 1295–1304* (Città del Vaticano, 1942), 2 vols. Unpublished sources include the 1427–28 tax returns of hospitals in the *Catasto* 185.11, 190, 194, 195, 291, 292, 293, and the 1495 tax returns in *Decima della Repubblica*, 66–70.

9. For population estimates of Florence see D. Herlihy and C. Klapisch-Zuber, *Les toscans et leurs familles. Une étude du catasto florentin de 1427* (Paris, 1978), 165–77, and wage rates R.A. Goldthwaite, *The Building of Renaissance Florence. An Economic and Social History* (Baltimore, London, 1980), 436–9.

10. See Herlihy and Klapisch, *Les toscans*, 176–7.

11. On the numbers of confraternities in Florence of this period

see J. Henderson, *Piety and Charity in Late-Medieval Florence*, Ch. 1 (forthcoming).

12. *Cronaca di Giovanni Villani a miglior lezione ridotta* (Florence, 1825), vol. 5, XI, xciv; C. Landino, *Scritti critici et teoretici*, ed. R. Cardini (Rome, 1974), vol. 1, 115.

13. Hospital returns appear in the following volumes of the *Catasto*: 185. 1–11; 190; 194.11; 195; 291; 292; 293; *Decima della repubblica* 66–70; for the 1527 census see Biblioteca Nazionale Centrale di Firenze (cited as BNF), NA 987.

14. On France see Michel Mollat's chapters in J. Imbert (ed.), *Histoire des hôpitaux en France* (Toulouse, 1982), and especially 35–47, 78–9; for Avignon see J. Chiffoleau, *La compatibilité de l'au-delà. Les hommes, la mort et la religion dans la région d'Avignon à la fin du moyen-age (vers 1320–vers 1480)* (Rome, 1980), 314–21; Genoa, C. Marchesini and G. Sperati, *Ospedali Genovesi nel medioevo. Atti della società Ligure di storia patria*, n.s. XXI (1981), 60–2; *contado* of Florence, C.M. de La Roncière, *Florence, centre économique regional au XIVe siècle* (Aix-en-Provence, 1976), 921–36; Milan, G. Albini, *Guerra, fame, peste. Crisi di mortalità e sistema sanitario nella Lombardia tardomedioevale* (Milan, 1982), 63–78.

15. This was also the case for Genoa (Marchesini and Sperati, 60–63), Lyon (N. Gonthier, *Lyon et ses pauvres au moyen-age (1350–1500)* (Lyon, 1978), 142), Toulouse (Imbert (ed.), *Histoire des hôpitaux*, p. 107), and London (C. Rawcliffe, 'The hospitals of late medieval London', *Medical History*, 28 (1984), 4–5). Pistoia, however, seems to have been somewhat exceptional with eleven hospitals for 4,500 inhabitants (D. Herlihy, *Medieval and Renaissance Pistoia. The Social History of an Italian Town* (New Haven, 1967), 247–8).

16. Their development is surveyed by Davidsohn, *Storia di Firenze* VII, 87–104, esp. 87–91.

17. Op. cit., 87–8.

18. Op. cit., 89.

19. ibid.

20. Villani, *Cronaca* XI, 94.

21. See the map showing the locations of the 'Principali ospedali dei secoli XIII e XIV' in the city of Florence in G. Fanelli, *Firenze. Le città nella storia d'Italia* (Rome-Bari, 1981 ed.), 49. See also the maps of Florence at the end of the last volume of W. and E. Paatz, *Die Kirchen von Florenz*.

22. Rubio Vela, *Podreza, enfermedad*, 26: Mollat, in Imbert (ed.), *Histoire des hôpitaux*, 100: G. Giordanego, 'Les hôpitaux arlésiens du XIIe au XIVe siècle', *Assistance et charité*, Cahiers de Fanjeaux, 13 (Toulouse,1978), 190–3.

23. Cf. also the discussion of the position of the Ospedale di S. Paolo in Goldthwaite and Rearick, 'Michelozzo and the Ospedale di San Paolo in Florence', 222–3.

24. On the building of the walls see G. Fanelli, *Firenze*, 35–7.

25. See de La Roncière, *Florence, centre économique*, 679–91.

26. See J. Henderson, 'Charity in late-medieval Florence: the role of religious confraternities', in *Florence and Milan. Acts of two conferences at Villa I Tatti in Florence*, 11 (Florence, 1988), 147–63.

27. P. Fanfani (ed.), *Capitoli della Compagnia dei Portatori o S. Giovanni Decollato* (Bologna, 1858), 9–10, 6–7.

28. On S. Paolo see Passerini, 163–88, Goldthwaite and Rearick, 'Michelozzo', and B.J. Trexler, 'Hospital patients'; S. Maria Nuova see Passerini, 284–395 and Pampaloni, *Lo spedale di Santa Maria Nuova*. Another substantial hospital, that of S. Gallo, had been founded in 1218: Passerini, 659–75 and R.C. Trexler, 'The foundlings of Florence, 1395–1455'.

29. Passerini, 835–6.

30. See J. Newton, 'Poverty and charity in late-medieval Florence' PhD dissertation (Brown University, Rhode Island, forthcoming). I am grateful to Jeffrey Newton for having given me the opportunity to read a draft version of his thesis.

31. On Orsanmichele see S. La Sorsa, *La compagnia d'Or S. Michele ovvero una pagina della beneficenza in Toscana nel secolo XIV* (Trani, 1955) and Henderson, *Piety and Charity*, Part 2.

32. In Florence the legal position of women is discussed by T. Kuehn, *Emancipation in Late-Medieval Florence* (New Brunswick, 1982) and 'Some ambiguities of female inheritance ideology in the Renaissance', *Continuity and Change*, 2 (1987), 11–36, as well as C. Klapisch-Zuber, *Women, Family and Ritual in Renaissance Italy* (Chicago and London, 1985), Ch. 6, 10. A number of Italian communes passed legislation protecting the rights of orphans and widows: for Florence see *Provvisioni registri* 36, f. 3r: 29 August 1348; for Milan, G.C. Bascapé, 'L'assistenza e la beneficenza a Milano dall'alto medioevo alla fine della dinastia sforzesca', *Storia di Milano* (Milan, 1957), VIII, 394; and for Orvieto, E. Carpentier, *Une ville devant la peste. Orvieto et la peste noire de 1348* (Paris, 1962), 146.

33. M. Villani, *Cronaca di Matteo Villani a miglior lezione ridotta* (Florence, 1825), 1, 1, vii.

34. *Provvisioni Registri* 36, f. 3r: 29 August 1348.

35. On the Orbatello see Passerini, 641, and R.C. Trexler, 'A widow's asylum of the Renaissance: the Orbatello of Florence', in P.N. Stearns (ed.), *Old Age in Pre-Industrial Society* (New York, 1982), 119–49; on the Innocenti see Passerini, 685, 704; on the Monte delle Doti see J. Kirschner and A. Molho, 'The dowry fund and the marriage market in early Quattrocento Florence', *Journal of Modern History*, 50 (1978), 403–38.

36. This is a theme of Mollat in Imbert (ed.), *Histoire des hôpitaux*, 130, and K. Park, 'Healing the poor: hospitals and medicine in renaissance Florence', an article which is forthcoming and conceived as complementary to the present paper.

37. M. Villani, *Cronaca*, 1, vii.

38. See S. Maria Nuova 1, f. 1r.

39. Passerini, 843.

40. Goldthwaite and Rearick, 'Michelozzo', 222–4.

41. Passerini, 150 and 223.

42. Passerini, 125–33.

43. *Catasto* 291, ff. 23^{r-v}; BNF, N.A. 987, f. 23^{v}.

44. D. Moreni (ed.), *Prediche del Beato Fra Giordano da Pisa dell'ordine dei predicatori recitati in Firenze dal MCCCIII al MCCCVI* (Florence, 1831), 1, 55. It is unclear from the first sentence ('Va' pure agli spedali, o cola a San Gallo') whether he is suggesting that these patients were from the Ospedale di S. Gallo or from other hospitals in Via S. Gallo. Although the Ospedale di S. Gallo is best known as an institution for foundlings, in the late thirteenth century it also catered for more general categories of poor people, as can be seen from a law of 19 May 1294, which refers to both paupers and infants: Passerini, 936.

45. B.J. Trexler, 'Hospital patients', 45–6, 53, and Park, 'Hospitals and medical welfare'.

46. For S. Maria della Scala see *Catasto* 185, ff. 584^{r}–585^{v}; S. Gallo, Passerini, 669; the Innocenti, Passerini, 704. For more details about the foundling hospitals see Trexler, 'The foundlings of Florence'.

47. Passerini, *Storia*, 106.

48. *Catasto* 185, f. 626^{r}: 'una vedova d'anni 80 ed è inferma e non escie di letto; una donna d'anni 25 è stata inferma un' anno o più e da infermità da non ghuarire mai sennone quando si morra di quello'.

49. *Cronaca di Giovanni Villani*, XI, 94.

50. Population estimates in Herlihy and Klapisch, *Les toscans* 177, 183.

51. Corsini, *La 'morìa'*, 34.

52. L.B. Alberti, *L'architettura* [De Re Aedificatoria], ed. G. Orlandi and P. Portoghesi (Milan, 1966), 1, 367–8.

53. On S. Maria della Scala see D. Gallavotti Cavallaro, *L'ospedale di S. Maria della Scala in Siena. Vicende di una committenza artistica* (Pisa, 1985); O. Redon, 'Autour de l'Hôpital Santa Maria della Scala à Sienne au XIIIe siècle', *Ricerche storiche*, XV (1985), 17–34; and S.R. Epstein, *Alle origini della fattoria toscana. L'ospedale della Scala di Siena e le sue terre (metà-'200-metà-'400)*, (Florence, 1987).

54. Foster, 'Per il disegno', 7.

55. F. Leverotti, 'L'ospedale senese di S. Maria della Scala in una relazione del 1456', *Bullettino senese di storia patria*, XCI (1984), 276–92.

56. Leverotti, 'L'ospedale senese', 278–83.

57. Antonio Averlino detto il Filarete, *Trattato di architettura*, eds A.M. Finoli and L. Grassi (Milan, 1972), 299 n. 1.

58. M. Lazzarini and A. Munoz, *Filarete, sculture e architetto del XV* (Rome, 1968), 186.

59. Recent formulations of this idea are in H.M. Colvin, D.R.

Ransome, and J. Summerson (eds), *The History of the King's Works* (London, 1975), 199, and M.O. Banzola, *L'Ospedale vecchio di Parma* (Parma, 1980), 45.

60. See Foster, 'Per il disegno', 4–7.

61. ibid. I am grateful for this suggestion to Patrick Sweeney, who is at present preparing a history of the architectural development of S. Maria Nuova.

62. Leverotti, 'L'ospedale senese', 280, n. 22.

63. Foster, 'Per il disegno', 7–8.

64. Leverotti, 'L'ospedale senese', 301; C. Landino's Commentary on Dante's *Divine Comedy*, quoted in Passerini, 301.

65. See Goldthwaite and Rearick, 'Michelozzo', 279–80.

66. The cloisters for the Florentine hospitals of S. Paolo, S. Maria Nuova, Messer Bonifazio, and S. Matteo are visible in their ground plans, which are reproduced in Goldthwaite and Rearick, 'Michelozzo', 228, 274, 276, and 277. The cloisters of S. Maria Maggiore of Milan can be seen clearly in Filarete's designs: Foster, 'Per il disegno', 1–22.

67. Leverotti, 'L'ospedale senese', 281–3; Passerini, 851-73.

68. Herlihy, *Medieval and Renaissance Pistoia*, pp. 247–8.

69. L. Arbib (ed.), *Storia fiorentina di Benedetto Varchi* (Florence, 1838–41), 2, 101. S. Maria Nuova's property is listed in *Catasto* 185.11, ff. 640^r–699^r.

70. G. Brucker , 'Urban parishes and their clergy in Quattrocento Florence: a preliminary "sondage"', *Renaissance Studies in Honor of Craig Hugh Smyth* (Florence, 1985), 1, 27, n. 21.

71. *Catasto* 194.11, f. 380^r; *Catasto* 292, ff. 230^v–232^v.

72. *Catasto* 291, ff. 72^r, 68^r.

73. *Catasto* 185.11, ff. 601^r–606^r; Brucker, 'Urban parishes', 27 n. 21.

74. *Catasto* 194.11, ff. 172^v, 646^v, and 610^{r-v}; on confraternities see Henderson, *Piety and Charity*, Ch. 2, Table 3.

75. See, for example, the property belonging to S. Maria Nuova in *Catasto* 185.11, ff. 640^r–699^r, and below for a discussion of S. Matteo's assets.

76. See G. Pinto, *La Toscana nel tardo medioevo. Ambiente, economia rurale, società* (Firenze, 1982), 247–329.

77. The shares of Florentine hospitals in the communal debt are listed among their assets in their *Catasto* returns, as for S. Matteo (*Catasto* 185.11, ff. 601^r–606^r), and the Ospedale degli Innocenti (*Catasto* 190, ff. 80^r–82^v).

78. Passerini, 335, and R.A. Goldthwaite, 'Local banking in Renaissance Florence', *Journal of European Economic History*, 14 (1985), 44–5.

79. Passerini, 335.

80. ibid.

81. See I. Chabot, 'Poverty and the widow in late medieval Florence', in J. Henderson (ed.), *Charity and the Poor in Medieval and*

Renaissance Europe, Continuity and Change, 3 (2) (1988), 291–311. This process may be seen, for example, in the *Catasto* return of the Ospedale di S. Maria della Scala in *Catasto* 185, ff. 528ʳ–575ᵛ, where a number of houses were listed as not providing any income because they were occupied for life by the inhabitant.

82. Some idea of, for example, S. Maria Nuova's finances after the Black Death can be gained from the hospital's account books: S. Maria Nuova 4,397–4,400 (Uscita, 1348–1353) and 4,401–4,403 (Entrata e Uscita, 1349–1352). The records of testaments, though not complete, are in S. Maria Nuova 59 for 1300–1500 and S. Maria Nuova 60 for 1340–1379. The history of S. Maria Nuova from its foundation up to the Black Death is dealt with by J. Newton in 'Poverty and charity'.

83. On S. Maria della Scala see Epstein, *Alle origini*.

84. *Catasto* 185.11, ff. 604ᵛ–605ʳ: 'Di tutti i sopra ditti debitori mai non se ne chavera uno denaio però chi è morto e chi se ne ito e chi fallito e di loro niente si truova . . . sichè anchora i sopradetti debitori si può dire siamo perduti.'

85. Herlihy, *Medieval and Renaissance Pistoia*, 247–8; *Catasto* 190, f. 83ʳ; 185, f. 619ʳ.

86. See the purchases of the Ospedale di S. Jacopo a S. Eusebio in *Catasto* 291, f. 23ʳ; S. Bonifazio, op. cit., ff. 33ᵛ–34ʳ. Examples of food purchases by S. Maria Nuova are contained in the Libri dell'Uscita for 1440–1 and 1456–8 (S. Maria Nuova 4,489 and 4,499).

87. Passerini, 305.

88. The duties of the staff of S. Maria Nuova are outlined in its early sixteenth-century ordinances: Passerini, 851–67. The accounts of S. Maria Nuova have been used by two economic historians to calculate wage-rates for skilled and unskilled labourers: de La Roncière, *Florence, centre économique*, and Goldthwaite, *The Building of Renaissance Florence*.

89. See Goldthwaite and Rearick; 'Michelozzo'; and Passerini 304–6.

90. *Catasto* 185.11, f. 613ʳ, Spedale di S. Antonio e S. Niccholo; f. 615ʳ, Spedale di San Giuliano; f. 617ʳ, Spedale di Sancto Lò; f. 629ʳ, Spedale di S. Maria al Merchatale della Scarperia. *Catasto* 293, f. 35ᵛ, Spedale di S. Maria dell'Umiltà; ibid., Spedale di San Lorenzo a San Piero Ghattolino; f. 56ʳ, Spedale di San Nicholò a San Felice in Piazza.

91. Passerini, 304–6.

92. Goldthwaite and Rearick; 'Michelozzo', 223; Passerini, 305.

93. *Catasto* 291, f. 34ʳ; 185.11, f. 606ᵛ; Passerini, 302, 305.

94. *Catasto* 185, f. 58ʳ.

95. K. Park, *Doctors and Medicine in Early Renaissance Florence* (Princeton, 1985), 157.

96. Passerini, 859.

97. Passerini, 859.

98. For more details see the ordinances themselves in Passerini, 858–61 and a fuller discussion of the medical aspects see the forthcoming article by Park, 'Healing the Poor: hospitals and medicine in renaissance Florence'.

99. Passerini, 865.

100. ibid.

101. B. Trexler, 'Hospital patients', 41–59, and Park, *Doctors and Medicine*, 106 and expanded in her forthcoming article 'Healing the poor: hospitals and medicine in renaissance Florence'.

102. The exceptions are the articles mentioned above by Goldthwaite and Rearick, Park, B.J. Trexler and R.C. Trexler.

103. See the speech delivered by Leonardo Bruni in favour of providing finance for the building of the Ospedale degli Innocenti in 1421: F. del Migliore, *Firenze, città nobilissima illustrata* (Florence, 1694), 307–9.

104. Friedenthal, *Luther*, p. 78.

105. Quoted in Passerini, 333.

106. On plague in Florence see M.S. Mazzi, 'La peste a Firenze nel quattrocento', in R. Comba, G. Piccini, and G. Pinto (eds), *Strutture familiari, epidemie e migrazioni nell'Italia medievale* (Naples, 1984), 91–115, and A.G. Carmichael, *Plague and the Poor in Renaissance Florence* (Cambridge, 1986).

107. On S. Maria Nuova, for example, see Passerini, 296–8, 300.

108. Corsini, *La 'morìa'*, 34.

109. ibid., and on the role of charitable institutions in Florence during subsequent epidemics see J. Henderson, 'Plague in Renaissance Florence: medical theory and government response', in N. Bulst, R. Delort (eds) *Maladies et Société* (XIIe–XVIIIe siècles) (Paris, 1988).

110. Corsini, *La 'morìa'*, p.34.

111. J.D. Thompson and G. Goldin, *The Hospital: A Social and Architectural History* (New Haven, London, 1975), 31.

112. Examples include Brescia, Bergamo, and Cremona: *Storia di Brescia* (Brescia, 1961), 1, 1,117–1,119; B. Pullan, *Rich and Poor*, 203–5; Foster, 'Per il Disegno', 8.

113. See A. d'Addario, *La formazione dello stato moderno in Toscana dal Cosimo il Vecchio a Cosimo I de'Medici* (Lecce, 1976), 243–5, and Passerini, 307–8.

4

Charity, power, and patronage in eighteenth-century Italian hospitals: the case of Turin

Sandra Cavallo

1

Recent research on the system of poor relief in Italy has largely overlooked the question of philanthropy, that is the involvement of the laity in managing and financing charitable institutions. Research on the English case has paid considerable attention to the role of private benefactors, prestige, social influence, and competition between individuals and groups via charitable actions. However, studies in the field in Italy, which emerged above all from the 1970s onwards, have tended to explain the evolution of the poor relief system almost entirely in terms of religious ideology and state policy. The church and state are held responsible for the transformation in the patterns of relief and care for the poor and sick from the fifteenth to the eighteenth century.

According to the standard chronology and interpretation, the religious and moral climate of the Catholic Reformation, and then Counter Reformation, brought about the boom in charitable initiatives designed for different categories of the needy from the late sixteenth to the early seventeenth century (these initiatives included provision for incurables, beggars, young women, prisoners, and prisoners condemned to the gallows). Although groups of lay people were the real creators of the dense network of charities set up over some 200 years, their activity is usually seen as driven by religious motivations; they are pictured as little more than the executors of the will of the Counter Reformation Church, and their behaviour is regarded as prompted by the preaching of the religious orders and the voice of the confessor.

The lack of interest amongst historians in the role of private charity is even clearer in the studies dealing with the period of absolutism. The control of the relief system is said to have been taken over by the state from the seventeenth century. The central authority is thought to have engaged in a comprehensive restructuring of the poor relief system in an effort to distinguish the deserving from the undeserving poor, and then to separate them through a series of measures, such as banishment and segregation. It is forgotten, however, that, even while the state's control over institutions was strengthened, private charity often remained the main source of finance for charitable provision.[1] Finally, the evolution of hospitals for the sick is seen as separate. The hospital's transformation from a 'general refuge' into a place devoted to sick care, with clinical and experimental functions, is usually linked to the Enlightenment reforms, which took place in a few Italian states in the late eighteenth century. In fact, the phenomenon is seen as restricted to those areas most affected by Enlightenment thought. Meanwhile, the persistence of the idea of the charitable vocation is seen as retarding the 'medicalization' of the Italian hospital well into the late nineteenth century.[2]

The scant attention given to lay involvement in charity, in my opinion, largely reflects shortcomings in methodology and approach rather than any peculiarity of the Italian model, i.e. the hypothesis of the predominance of centralization over charitable activities. Indeed, the tendency to attribute the development of the charity system to impersonal forces seeking ideological and social control has meant ignoring the actions of real social subjects and neglecting their motivations. It is not, therefore, by chance that the most valuable sources for documenting the aims and functions of charitable provision, the social groups involved, and the systems of power at work have been largely disregarded by recent histories; the minute books, the records of recipients and patients, budgets, donations, and wills have largely gone unconsulted.

My research has pursued a different approach in seeking to identify *who* managed the provision for the poor and sick, and to analyse the social characteristics of benefactors, governors, and recipients. It has aimed to throw light on the motivations guiding philanthropy and the social meaning of various forms of poor relief. Charitable activity has therefore been examined in the wider context: first, of relationships within the local elites, connecting different influence groups; and, second, the vertical ties joining the ruling social groups and the labouring classes. The picture which emerges from this reconstruction differs at important points from the normal representation of the poor and sick relief systems. Above all, explanations based on the concepts of social control and religious sentiment are shown to be inadequate, while the part played by private initiative turns out to be crucial. Moreover, the trends in development and characteristics of charity appear deeply rooted in the local dynamics of protection, patronage, and social conflict.

My argument will be mostly grounded in the findings of research on the operation of the charity system in Turin, the capital of the Savoy Kingdom, during the eighteenth century. This case is especially interesting in that the Savoyard state has frequently been described as an example of absolutism and marked centralization, from the time of the reforms of Victor Amadeus II from 1680 to 1730, later consolidated by his successor. The poor relief system is usually regarded as a 'creation' of the absolute monarchy, as embodied by the celebrated measures of 1717 designed to eradicate begging and pauperism by setting up a network of hospitals and charities in every part of the kingdom.[3]

Turin, which was the centre of court life and state administration, also became the principal manufacturing centre of the kingdom in the last quarter of the seventeenth century. Its industrial structure, hingeing mainly on silk manufacture, was further reinforced in the following century. A consequence of this (together with demographic growth and the concentration of landed property) was that the city attracted more and more people from the countryside, doubling its size during the eighteenth century, from 45,000 to 90,000 inhabitants.

I will begin this article by broadly outlining the structure of charitable provision in the capital in the eighteenth century, underlining some of the features common to the systems of relief in Italy under the *ancien régime*. I will then focus on the main hospital for the sick in Turin, and follow its development from the late seventeenth century, dealing in particular with the consequences for the hospital's functioning

arising from the shift to state control and to closer links with
the medical faculty established during the eighteenth century.

2

By the eighteenth century, charitable aid to the sick was concentrated in just two hospitals: the Hospital of San Giovanni,
which was very old and had from 1440 been the city's
principal hospital following the incorporation of twelve small
medieval hospitals that were located near the main access
roads into Turin; and, second, the Hospital of San Maurizio
and Lazzaro, which was established in 1575 at the initiative
of the knightly order of that name.[4] The Hospital of San
Giovanni, originally administered by the Metropolitan
Chapter and put under the jurisdiction of the bishop, passed
into the hands of a mixed administration in 1541. The city
council saved the hospital from a crisis following a long
period of invasions, plague, and famine, and, in exchange,
took a role in the hospital's administration. From then on,
the board of governors was always made up of four city coun-
cillors and four canons from the Metropolitan Church. So,
here we have an authority with a strong civic identity, the
expression of the local oligarchy, and independent of central
control. The case of the Hospital of San Maurizio and
Lazzaro was different. While under the administration of a
military order subject to the sovereign, it was within the
sphere of influence of an aristocracy whose powers extended
beyond the confines of the city, as well as being tied to the
court and military authority. It was no coincidence that the
Hospital of San Maurizio and Lazzaro received handsome
endowments from the sovereign, while that of San Giovanni
was economically self-reliant.

The way in which the particular institutions belonged to
different social contexts and areas of influence is clear at first
glance, and this seems to have been a characteristic of the
organization of relief until the late eighteenth century; that is,
until these spheres of influence were swept away and the
management of the institutions passed into the hands of state
officials. Even the governing body of the Ospedale di Carità,
Turin's large centre for poor relief, strongly reflected a
particular social milieu – that of the mercantile and industrial

elites. If we bear in mind that the majority (over 40 per cent) of those helped by the hospital were artisans, it is evident that the governor's post was a highly influential one, and enabled bankers, merchants, and masters to control the distribution of relief to the urban working population and industrial sectors in crisis, correcting imbalances in the labour market.

The charitable institutions in Turin seem to have had a defined function from the time of their origin. For example, the Hospitals of San Maurizio and San Giovanni were designed for the sick from the time of their foundation. In consequence, we have not come across cases which evoke the image of the 'refuge for all' often referred to. Previously, the Hospital of San Giovanni had also occasionally played the role of assisting the poor, above all by distributing bread and money rather than by providing shelter.[5] However, such functions were soon assumed by the Ospedale di Carità, a poorhouse founded in 1627 by a private benefactor, though not properly operational until 1649 (due to plague and war interrupting), and not so large until the move to a new site in 1682.

The Ospedale di Carità is one of the number of hospitals for the poor and for beggars set up during two bouts of hospital founding in several Italian cities at the end of the sixteenth and at the end of the seventeenth centuries. Historians have usually pointed to the common set of factors behind the initiatives, through which a new model of relief provision was supposed to have taken shape on the basis of separating 'genuine' and 'false' beggars, and subjecting the latter through repression and segregation. Within an Italian context, the Ospedale di Carità in Turin is often considered to exemplify the procedure of *renfermement*, following the 1717 edicts outlawing begging in the kingdom. However, the hospital's records of recipients and registers of admission, along with other documents, throw a different light on the matter. The violent repression of begging via arrest and punishment seem, instead, to have been of marginal significance in the hospital's overall activities, and was resorted to only in moments of acute crisis, serving as a deterrent against the immigrants who used then to flock into the city. However, the majority of the inmates were admitted on a voluntary basis – up to 2,000 of them in crises. They included the single old people unable to work, and the legitimate children of large families who were left in the hospital's care for a limited period. Moreover, the inmates did not belong to marginal groups, but to the productive and established sections of the city economy. In fact, relief was restricted to those born or long resident in the city. Rather than being a place for the detention of beggars, the Ospedale di Carità seems to have been a centre for relief on which the working population depended for its subsistence strategies.[6]

The system for selection of supplicants judged worthy to receive relief was rigorous. The poor were examined in person by a delegation of governors who required the presence of the whole family of supplicants. They checked not only their citizenship qualifications, but whether they were able to work, whether they were genuinely sick (as certified by a physician or surgeon), and the proportion of bread-winners to the number of mouths to be fed in a family unit. The relief given was often a combination of different kinds, ranging from the admittance of old people and children aged 7 to 14 to payment for wet-nursing newborn infants and the weekly distribution of a fixed quantity of bread.

The selection of supplicants was, therefore, carried out on the basis of criteria designed to differentiate the poor according to their degree of need. Nevertheless, it is clear that other factors entered into the decision as to who was eligible for relief – factors like status, protection, and the capacity certain groups had to bring pressure to bear. An obvious case in point is the favour that was invariably extended to the domestics of the more distinguished families. As for artisans, some trades were better protected because of the power of parts of the merchant and industrial elites, who, of course, were often represented on the board of governors of the hospital. Relief was only to a limited extent given on an equitable basis. Historians have generally held up the distinction made between the 'deserving' and 'undeserving' poor as an important step in the development of more rational forms of relief – that is, when it ceased to be given universally and indiscriminately as required by the Christian ideal, and became a social action. However, we should not forget that the category of 'deserving' poor was only partly moral and economic. Apart from degree of need, this category amply reflected the configurations of privilege and protection that were found among the poor.

The link between relief and privilege is, of course, a characteristic of charity in an *ancien régime* type of society. This becomes especially clear if we examine several forms of relief found in pre-industrial European societies. Take, for example, the secret relief given to the 'shamefaced poor' (*poveri vergognosi*), who did not dare to beg since they had fallen from a higher social station; or the dowry funds and institutions created for girls of respectable family origins; or the relief reserved for specific professional groups. These appear to be initiatives that helped relieve a kind of poverty that we can call 'relative' – relative, that is, to status, family of origin, to the style of living considered appropriate to the social or professional group to which the needy person belonged. These initiatives were found in Spain, France, and in many Italian states, though in seventeenth and eighteenth century England they survived only in the form of relief reserved for members of craft companies or specific national groups.[7]

Recent historical research inspired by Foucault's work has tended to deal with large institutions, overlooking these activities, and considering them obsolete remnants of Counter-Reformation forms of charity.[8] Yet their scale was anything but insignificant, and often accounted for a high percentage of money paid out in charity. In Turin, the Compagnia di San Paolo had, in the eighteenth century, a budget equivalent to that of the Hospital of San Giovanni or the Ospedale di Carità, for three purposes: the administration of dowry funds; for the shamefaced poor; and for the women's institutions. In Naples, lay groups distributed 655 dowries and helped approximately 5,000 persons in thirty-nine institutions in one year alone in the seventeenth century. These included *conservatori* for young women, institutions for the young and aged, and hospitals reserved for the 'relative poor' (those belonging to specific social or professional groups, such as craft companies, employees in public administration, the army). Furthermore, these practices did not die out, but continued to thrive in the next century. The institutions for women went on sprouting in the eighteenth century, so that by the 1800s there were at least eighty of them. Likewise, in Rome and Turin four new institutions were added to the existing three.[9] Although these *conservatori* or *ricoveri* for women have been described as typical expressions of Counter-Reformation thinking designed to defend female honour and prevent sinfulness, the timing of their development seems to contradict this interpretation. Even relief for the shamefaced poor, usually considered a sixteenth-century phenomenon, develops at different times in different situations. This form of relief developed in Venice in the sixteenth century, in Bologna in the following century, and became particularly important in Turin in the mid eighteenth century.[10]

What then was the significance of these initiatives? Despite the variations in chronology, these different forms of charity seem to have shared a common goal; namely, the defence of the prestige and image of the social group to which the recipient of charity belonged via measures to arrest the decline of individuals and families. For instance, the dowry subsidy, one of the most widespread forms of relief, allowed respectable families in economic difficulties to marry off their daughters to a person of similar rank. The dowry allowed them to maintain the name and honour of the family, and, at the same time, reaffirmed the dignity of the social group and lines of demarcation between the social classes.

The measures for the relief of 'relative' poverty, which were common in *ancien-régime* societies, appear, therefore, to have corresponded to the need to reaffirm or redefine the hierarchical social order. It did so by upholding the prestige of an old or new elite – an acutely felt need when new social groups were emerging. Hence, the unevenness of developments, even within the Italian context. It could be suggested that, as a general rule, the importance of these forms of charity was strictly related to whether a period was stable or marked by major upheavals in the social order. We can see in the Turin case that a visible increase in measures to help the shamefaced poor (together with dowry funds and the creation of new institutions for women) correlates with a phase of conflict and social change in which the hereditary and court nobility's loss of status coincided with the emergence of a new class of officials who pressed for public recognition and marks of prestige. In 1734 the latter obtained a revision of the category 'shamefaced' poor; it was redefined so that it included not only 'nobles by birth' and 'those nobles so declared by the royal sovereign', but also 'all those rendered noble by their profession'. In effect, this encompassed almost the entire state bureaucratic class, right down to the lowest rungs of the professional and military ladder.[11] Even the merchant classes in this period managed to have the privilege extended to its members with the establishment of a fund for the 'shamefaced poor of the second class'; a fund, that is, for merchants, shopkeepers, and bankers, 'to the exclusion of the nobility'.[12] So, the investment on behalf of the 'relative' poor was not limited to a purely defensive need to conserve social status pursued by social groups threatened by the rise of new elites. It also represented a means of achieving upward mobility. In mid-eighteenth century Turin a desire for symbolic recognition of gains made pushed the emerging classes to invest in these forms of 'privileged' charity. Redefining who was deemed worthy of receiving special types of relief entailed reflecting and sanctioning changes that had taken place in the assignation of prestige.

There is not space here to provide a detailed reconstruction of the transformations affecting the make-up of the elites in Turin at the time. Yet it is worth noting how the re-ordering of the configurations of power at the top of the social hierarchy was also reflected in the criteria regulating the provision of charity. In the second half of the eighteenth century, if a family included a state employee among its members, it had a far better chance of gaining access to relief provision. As we have already mentioned in relation to the relief provided by the Ospedale di Carità, the category of the 'deserving poor' was fluid and ill-defined, and acquired different meanings depending on the model of protection in a particular social context.

3

The extent and significance of the laity's role in the poor relief institutions can best be appreciated if we examine a particular example. For Turin, a good case to take is the Hospital of San Giovanni, the largest hospital for the sick in the city. For a long time, the Hospital of San Giovanni remained a modest institution with only thirty-six beds (half for men and half for women), in the middle of the seventeenth

Table 4.1 Endowments of beds for incurables and curables from private benefactors at the Hospital of San Giovanni, 1668–1790.

No. of beds		No. of beds		No. of beds		No. of beds	
Year Inc.	Cur.	Year Inc.	Cur.	Year Inc.	Cur.	Year Inc.	Cur.
1668 2	–	1700 2	–	1732 4	–	1764 1	–
1669 –	–	1701 3	–	1733 –	–	1765 1	2
1670 2	–	1702 –	–	1734 4	–	1766 –	–
1671 1	–	1703 2 + u	–	1735 8	2 + u	1767 –	–
1672 –	–	1704 1	1	1736 2	–	1768 1	–
1673 –	–	1705 1	1	1737 1	–	1769 –	–
1674 –	–	1706 –	–	1738 2	–	1770 –	–
1675 –	–	1707 –	–	1739 5	–	1771 3	–
1676 1	–	1708 –	1	1740 4	–	1772 –	–
1677 2	–	1709 3	2	1741 4	–	1773 2	–
1678 7	–	1710 1	–	1742 –	–	1774 1*	–
1679 1	–	1711 12	–	1743 3 + u	–	1775 1	–
1680 4	–	1712 9	–	1744 1	–	1776 –	14
1681 u	–	1713 4	–	1745 1	–	1777 1	–
1682 3	20	1714 4	1	1746 3	–	1778 –	–
1683 2	–	1715 2	–	1747 5	–	1779 –	–
1684 2	–	1716 1	–	1748 2	–	1780 –	3
1685 2	–	1717 2	1	1749 1	–	1781 –	–
1686 –	–	1718 1	2	1750 4	–	1782 –	1
1687 2	–	1719 2	–	1751 1	–	1783 1	–
1688 2	–	1720 2	1	1752 3	40	1784 2	2
1689 1	–	1721 1	–	1753 –	–	1785 –	1
1690 –	2	1722 –	–	1754 4	1	1786 –	1 + u
1691 3	–	1723 1	–	1755 7	–	1787 –	7
1692 –	–	1724 –	–	1756 2	1	1788 –	–
1693 2	–	1725 2	–	1757 3	–	1789 –	2 + u
1694 1	–	1726 –	–	1758 4	–	1790 –	1
1695 3	–	1727 –	–	1759 2	–		
1696 –	–	1728 2	–	1760 21*			
1697 1	–	1729 1	–	1761 –	–		
1698 1	–	1730 5	–	1762 1	2		
1699 –	–	1731 6	1	1763 2*	–		

Inc. = incurables   Cur. = curables

The dates refer to the moment of the disposition, which does not always coincide with that of the setting up of beds (see note 14 at end of chapter). Sometimes the testator did not indicate the exact number of beds but stated that as many as the estate permitted be established (usually the choice was between one or two), once the debts and other dispositions had been taken care of. In this case the letter 'u' (undetermined) appears in the table. The asterisk indicates the acquisitions of rights of nomination for beds existing already (see note 19 at end of chapter).

century. Its expansion began in 1668 when a new ward for the chronically ill was opened, the Opera Incurabili. The need for this ward had been discussed for a couple of years by the civic authorities and representatives of the various charities.[13] Unfortunately, the records of these discussions have not survived, but perhaps one of the factors that motivated the hospital's decision was that a ward for incurables would attract private donors. This, in any case, was the effect.

The endowment of a bed for incurables (via the payment of 5,200 lire until 1752, when the sum was increased to 6,250 lire) gave the benefactor and the persons he designated his successors (normally his descendants in the direct male line, or in the female line if there were no males) the perpetual right to select an incurable patient who would occupy the bed until his death. This new form of charity guaranteed the donor and his family direct and perpetual control over the use of the endowment, and this probably explains the very substantial growth in bequests and donations which the hospital received after the foundation of the new ward. It was, above all, this form of endowment which allowed the hospital to increase its capacity to around 220 curables and incurables in 1730, reaching 450 in 1792. Over 177 beds for incurables were set up by private benefactors between 1668, when the new ward was established, and 1754, when the board of governors started to restrict such endowments to encourage benefactors to found beds for curables instead. Despite these restrictions, another twenty-nine beds for incurables were endowed between 1754 and 1780.[14]

The number of beds for curables grew much more slowly. There were only fifty-eight beds for curables and twenty for convalescents given by private donors by 1754 (see Table 4.1). Furthermore, it should be noted that these seventy-eight beds were set up thanks to the generous donations from just two benefactors – the Marquis Villa (twenty beds for convalescents given in 1752) and Costeis, the banker, (forty beds for curables given in 1752). In the space of some eighty years or so, a total of only seventeen donors chose this form of charity, as against 114 who set up one or more beds for incurables. The benefactors' preference aggravated the imbalance between beds available for the sick and the increasing number available for incurables. The latter were soon as numerous as the former, and sometimes more so.

There were times in the eighteenth century when the board of governors was itself able to set up some beds for the curably sick, since the hospital's finances were in a healthy state; in 1713, six were set up, in 1723, another six, and then fifty in 1724.[15] Meanwhile, during the drawn-out economic crisis of 1734-50, due to famine, war, and epidemics, the hospital had to weather serious financial difficulties, added to, as we shall see, by imprudent policies foisted on the governors by government officials. The biggest burden of all was the building of the grandiose cross-shaped edifice that was supposed to serve as a new site for the Hospital of San Giovanni. For nearly a hundred years, from 1680 onwards, this absorbed most of the hospital's income, for although the board of governors had received the land as a gift from the Regent, it had to pay for all the building by itself.

It is true that beds for incurables were eventually turned into beds for the curable sick. The formula used for the endowment prescribed that when the founder's line of descent died out, the bed reverted to the board of governors, who had the power to change it into a bed for curables. This did increase provision for the sick, but only very gradually. Set up as one of the hospital wards, the Opera Incurabili had grown in a quite unforeseen way. The hospital was filled with old people and invalids whom the staff could do little for. In theory, the endowment conditions specified that persons nominated for a place as an incurable had to be examined by the hospital physician or surgeon to see whether they were really afflicted by an incurable disease.[16] In practice, however, the physician's opinion more often than not obsequiously concurred with the choice made by the donors, who were the hospital's principal benefactors. The incurables were, in consequence, the elderly governess and the coachman of the donor families, or persons who formed part of the protection network of these families, and so were provided with some insurance against old age.

The defects of this system did not escape observers at the time. As early as 1734, in a discussion of the measures to take in order to reorganize the city's poor relief structure, which had been under pressure in the wake of economic depression and epidemics, a complaint was made about the ward for incurables; it was said not to lack bequests, but

> in the name of being incurable . . . persons are accepted
> who are invalids rather than sick ranging from old age,
> blindness, lameness and other reasons, and are rightfully
> the responsibility of the Ospedale di Carità . . . since
> they have no need of any treatment for their ills, but
> only of food to satisfy their hunger.

In order to get the hospital to 'carry out its purpose, that is, to provide for the sick', it was suggested – without saying how – that the rules concerning the private nomination of patients be changed.[17] It is worth noting that the observer in question, the Prince of Francavilla, was himself a distinguished benefactor of the hospital. In 1725, he endowed some seven beds for incurables left to the hospital in his mother's will in 1711, and in 1731 he added two more beds to those already controlled by the family. Despite the strictures he expressed in his role as a state official, as a member of one of the wealthiest families in Turin he did not shun the advantages and influence that control of beds for incurables brought – as a source of prestige and a resource used to reward the fidelity of those under his protection.

In effect, benefactors continued to prefer this form of charity to the free bequest. For much of the century, the board of governors was not able to stop or regulate a practice that had attracted most of the donations and bequests enjoyed by the hospital. In 1744, for example, it was calculated that four out of five bequests (coming to a total of 214,945 lire) left to the hospital from 1729 were earmarked for the foundation of beds for incurables, while only one in four were free bequests.[18] So, on the one hand, measures were taken in 1754 and 1773 to limit the period of control over the nomination of patients, and in 1762 they went as far as to prohibit the acceptance of further endowments. Yet, when money was needed, the governors resorted to this means which they knew would procure funds from the public.[19] Finally, in 1780, even given the decrease in the number of foundations of beds for incurables (these being unwillingly accepted by the board of governors), the number of beds for curables that were founded still did not increase, and the existing provision fell well short of demand. It was therefore decided to grant the right of nomination for beds for curables as well.[20] The benefactors thus gained control over ordinary patients' access to the hospital, just as in the English voluntary hospital, where patients were admitted with a letter of recommendation. But, strangely enough, the measure existed on paper without having practical effect. After 1780, the right of nomination was not conceded to any of the new founders, except for the stipulation that the initial occupant of the bed would be nominated by the benefactor, after which the bed would be free. In practice, the beds were used for some years for incurable patients (even if the term 'incurable' was no longer mentioned), and they were then made available to the curable patients. So, beds remained under the control of the health personnel, as had previously been the case.

We do not know whether the physicians had a direct part in preventing the 1780 ordinance from being carried out. The fact is that the change that this made was alien to the way in which access to the hospital had been administered for over 200 years. In addition, the key role physicians had traditionally played was reinforced during the eighteenth century. Although the hospital's financial dependence on private charity had permitted the benefactor effectively to privatize a ward, using it for exercising influence, the Hospital of San Giovanni became neither a shelter for all and sundry nor a hospital for the care of the chronically sick. The ward for curables continued to be run by the medical staff and supervised by the board of governors. As we shall see, it can be taken as an early example of 'medicalization'.

If I have spent some time discussing the situation of beds for incurables, it is in order to demonstrate the inadequacy of the stereotypical notions of irrationality or religious motivation usually employed to explain Catholic charity. This is further confirmed if we examine the history of the bequests for beds. In the seventeenth century, the number of bequests did not increase in the climate created by baroque *pietas* and the devotion engendered by the Counter Reformation, nor did they decline in the subsequent century of 'dechristianization'.[21] Bequests grew in the mid-eighteenth century – the 'secular' years in which the absolute state was consolidated (see Table 4.2). If anything, trends registered the most acute phases in the conflict between elites and in the

Table 4.2 Endowments of beds
for incurables per
decade

Year	No. of beds
1668–77	8
1678–87	23 + u
1688–97	13
1698–1707	10 + u
1708–17	38
1718–27	9
1728–37	33
1738–47	28 + u
1748–57	27
1758–67	9 + 23*
1768–77	8 + 1*
1778–87	3
1788–97	4

See Table 4.1 for explanatory notes.

reordering of the social hierarchy. In fact, philanthropy boomed precisely in those decades which saw the climax in the conflict between the court and feudal interests, the new stratum of officials (who were then busy taking over control of the various city institutions and spheres of influence), and the merchant class which was especially determined to establish areas of control free from bureaucratic interference. This complex confrontation between the social groups was symbolically embodied, as we have seen, in the conflict over who was entitled to be called a member of the shamefaced poor.

Between 1720 and 1760, sizeable bequests gave the city new institutions: a ward for patients with contagious diseases (previously untreated by hospitals) at the Ospedale di Carità in 1733; an institution for fallen women, built in 1747. In addition, funds earmarked for the 'relative' poor were increased via dowries and alms, as well as other initiatives. In this period an unprecedented sum was spent on charity. In relation to the Hospital of San Giovanni, it was the appearance on the scene of merchants, bankers, and shopkeepers as founder of beds for incurables (previously the reserve of those with court connections) that explains the increase in bequests that took place. The merchant classes were able to break the court monopoly on beds for incurables by systematically making bequests, so that over a few years the control of some fifty-six beds (thirty-five of which were in the hands of six families) were held by seventeen families.

It seems that philanthropy was inspired by profoundly secular aspirations and marked by rational calculation, even when the aims did not overlap with the interests of the sick and poor. The factors of prestige, influence and competition between social groups provide the best explanation for the trends in charitable donations. However, we should also consider the specific economic interests at work. If we examine the forms taken by charitable donations and the tenor of the contracts defining the terms of the agreement between the hospital and the benefactor, we can see how the act of charity was not always a one-way process, but often involved a more complex exchange in which the benefactor obtained (in return for his benefactions) the privilege of taking advantage of the availability of loans and investment opportunities offered by the hospital.

The development of the hospital's financial activities appears to have been connected with the project for a new hospital and the exceptional need for money that thereby ensued. Indeed, by the 1670s, the minutes of the board of governors' meetings were taken up with reports about credit and lending operations carried out with private individuals. Charity played a key role in those operations. The most common went as follows. The benefactor, while still alive, donated capital that after his death (and sometimes of others named) was used for charitable purposes, usually the setting up of beds for incurables. Meanwhile, a return (generally of 3–5 per cent of the capital invested, that is, the legal rate of interest) was paid annually during the lifetime of the benefactor or other persons designated in the will. The age of the donors, which tended to be fairly advanced, and the speed with which the hospital's obligations would be expedited figured highly in the calculations of the board of governors. These factors probably also served to establish the rate of interest. From the donor's point of view, such forms of charity largely represented an investment underwritten by the worthiness of the institution with whom the agreement was reached.

In this period, it should be noted, the opportunities for investing liquid assets were limited and full of risk. There was no banking system in the Savoyard state open to private investors, and savers were reluctant to lend to private banks because of their high failure rate; in fact, these banks dealt almost entirely with commercial credit.[22] The most common forms of investment were, therefore, the acquisition of credits. The main forms were: *censi* (guaranteed by income from property, land, and taxes); *tassi* (taxes owed by the communities); and the *Luoghi dei Monti di San Giovanni Battista* (shares of the public debt). Clearly, the annual income that could be obtained from the hospital was much less risky than the *censi*, which were invariably paid late, or the taxes, which often went uncollected (especially in times of war or bad harvests), while the issue of the *Luoghi dei monti*, which were much sought after by private individuals, were limited and insufficient to cover the demands of those with liquid capital to spare.

The shortcomings of the credit system meant that the Hospital of San Giovanni (as well as other charitable institutions, such as the Compagnia di San Paolo and the Ospedale di Carità) assumed an important role in the city economy, becoming an integral part of the financial structure. The hospital then reinvested the capital brought in, partly in land purchases, partly in other fixed assets, but above all it loaned considerable sums of money, usually at the legal interest rate of 3–5 per cent. In fact, a great number of private individuals turned to the hospital in search of an alternative to the normal high-interest loans. These transactions accounted for the major part of the hospital budget. In fact, only some 30 per cent of income came from rents from the institutions' properties and farms. The rest, apart from the small contribution made by alms and the foundlings' manufactures, came from its activities as a creditor.

Charity had become part and parcel of these financial dealings. A kind of exchange was undertaken between people who were either looking for a way of investing their money or for a loan on good terms, and the governors of the hospital, who were looking for ways to finance the institution. From the hospital's point of view, the profit did not flow so much from the difference between the interest on payments and withdrawals, as from the charitable gifts that formed the precondition for gaining entry to the hospital's system of credit. In 1735, for example, the board of governors granted a loan at 4 per cent interest to the Prince of Francavilla with the following words:

Although given the money shortage and the circumstances of the present war, the hospital could derive 5 or
even 6 per cent interest from a sum of 24,500 *lire*, since
it concerns a family so beneficent towards the hospital [it
had already founded nine beds for incurables], and so
that the undertaking is completely secure, the Board has
agreed to the request.[23]

Part of the advantages secured from agreements with the
hospital was then paid back in bequests and donations.
However, unlike the case with the high interest paid to a
moneylender, it did not involve a payment with no returns,
but, as we have seen with the beds for incurables, an investment accruing prestige and powers of patronage.

4

The existence of a large ward for incurable patients seems
once again to conjure up an image of the hospital-as-shelter
projected by historians, who refer to the Italian case in terms
of retarded 'medicalization'. However, if we analyse the ways
in which the ward for curables was traditionally run, then the
Hospital of San Giovanni appears in a very different light as
a forerunner in providing treatment of the sick. As a docu-
ment of 1541 tells us, the hospital physician or surgeon had,
from the sixteenth century, been doing visiting rounds of
patients twice a day on a regular basis.[24] From the second
half of the seventeenth century, if not earlier, the duties of
the dresser (according to the chief surgeon's instructions)
were carried out by the younger surgeons resident in the
hospital. Originally, there were three of them, but their
number increased steadily, reaching thirteen by the 1730s, to
keep pace with the increase in beds. These surgeons were
assisted with simple duties by a group of nurses, who were
drawn from the ranks of ex-foundlings taken back by the
hospital. Moreover, in the late seventeenth century, a private
benefactor donated funds to create the post of assistant
hospital physician, which was reserved for a young man, who
had worked full time in residence in the hospital, 'to observe
the progress of diseases and report on them to the chief
physician'. Both the positions of dresser and assistant hospital

physician were occupied by young surgeons who wanted to enter the profession, not by apprentices or students. They were initially directly employed by the board of governors for a year, with the chance of having their period of service extended if they proved suitable.[25]

The hospital, therefore, already had a teaching function well before the university reforms completed between 1720 and 1739 made it compulsory for students of medicine and surgery to spend time in hospital as a precondition for entry into the profession. Judging by the number of candidates applying for this kind of practical experience, the post must have been considered prestigious and a good addition to the *curriculum vitae*. As it happened, some young physicians, after a long stint in the hospital, obtained important appointments, like that of chief regimental surgeon or even chief surgeon in the Hospital of San Giovanni. Many acquired more modest positions in the army medical service, and a great number went out to practice in the provinces. The chief physician and surgeon of the hospital were, as a matter of course, very prominent figures in Piedmontese medical circles. For instance, they usually held the chair of Practical and Theoretical Medicine at the university, and, in the case of surgeons, they held the office of anatomist. Some were even court physicians, but these duties normally passed to the physicians of the Hospital of San Maurizio and Lazzaro. So, even before the reforms, informal but solid ties existed between the Hospital of San Giovanni and the university.

It is worth noting that it was the board of governors that controlled the hiring of dressers and physicians and made sure that they carried out their duties as stipulated. They also took disciplinary measures in cases of irregularity or remissness. Certainly the opinions of the chief physician and surgeon had a significant bearing on the choice of dressers and medical assistants, who were often the physicians' pupils and sometimes even their relatives. One Alberto Verna, for example, who held the post of chief physician at the Hospital of San Giovanni for over forty years (serving seven as a dresser), established a veritable dynasty inside the institution. Two nephews succeeded him in his post, in 1739 and then in 1752, after long periods as his assistants, while a third nephew became assistant physician earlier in 1712. However, on paper, every decision on the various aspects of the

111

hospital's life remained firmly in the hands of the governors; that is until the 1730s, when the authority of the board of governors became the object of fierce attacks. The attacks do not seem to have come so much from physicians demanding greater autonomy as from centralizers.

The governors' authority was also strengthened by life appointment, cut short only in cases of sickness necessitating resignation. So, we have examples of governors who managed hospital affairs for twenty or thirty years. As a rule the governors were regular in their attendance of board meetings, and carried out their duties with diligence. There were few cases of absenteeism or figurehead governors.

This, then, was more or less how hospitals worked and were managed when the university reforms transformed the system and syllabus of teaching, affecting the activities of the Hospital of San Giovanni too. As far as the Faculty of Medicine was concerned, the period of study was lengthened to five years, in line with the more established Faculties of Law and Theology. Particular importance was attached to practical medicine, which took up three of the five years' study. In addition, the students were required to follow demonstrations on cadavers and to attend hospital in the last two years of study. During this period, students would have received lessons at the patients' bedside and would have discussed the illnesses under observation and the most interesting cases in weekly meetings. Only those who had then been awarded a degree could practise medicine, and then only on completing two additional years of training with a hospital or an accredited physician. However, the most innovative of the reforms concerned surgery, which, from 1721, became a university faculty. The length of time studying was originally set at three years, but was lengthened to five years in line with the courses of the other faculties in 1738. For the students of surgery, too, practical experience in the Hospital became a crucial element in the curriculum.[26]

Consequently, the reforms made it clear that the hospital was a privileged place with regard to the teaching and research in medicine by greatly increasing the number of medical and surgical students in the hospital and requiring and making it compulsory for the hospital physicians to be members of the university faculty. Yet these reforms did not completely change the identity of the hospital, since, as we have seen, it was already carrying out the functions of training and maintaining the profession, even if in a minor capacity.

It is interesting to note how the Savoyard reforms came several decades before the better-known reforms in Tuscany and Lombardy that are usually seen as exemplifying and pioneering reform in Italy. Furthermore, it is worth pointing out that these Savoyard reforms were carried out despite the absence of Enlightenment influences, and, instead, constituted a step in the construction of the absolute state. The Turinese case disproves the argument, according to which hospitals with 'modern' features developed in Italy thanks largely to the Enlightenment-inspired reforms of the late eighteenth century. Greater weight should, instead, be attached to the hypothesis advanced by some scholars suggesting continuity in the Italian tradition in which the hospital was used as a place of research, teaching, and medical practice. According to them, the Morgagni clinic had its roots in a practice started in Italian hospitals in the early sixteenth century.[27]

As for hospital life, the real effects of the reforms were political. They served as a vehicle for launching a violent assault on the historical independence of the Hospital. These reforms allowed state officials to extend their spheres of influence in the Hospital and progressively usurp the traditional powers of the governors. In the 1750s, after more than twenty years of conflict between the board of governors and the central authorities, state officials became members of the board itself.

This conflict had already begun to raise its head before the reforms shook the hospital. In fact, in 1728 a project presented as the King's personal wish was proposed to the board of governors. It concerned the establishment of a maternity ward and a school of midwifery under the direction of a French midwife, who had undertaken training in Paris for the purpose. The project sounded to the governors like an unprecedented and aggressive intrusion of royal power into the administration of the hospital, and provoked a strong reaction on the part of the governors. They tried several times through representations to the King and his representative to have the project disowned. The clash took a violent turn, with the governors appealing to the Hospital's tradition of independence, and the central government representatives insisting that the wishes of the sovereign be respected. In the end, an investigation was set up on the Senate's orders to establish the origins of the charity and whether the Hospital should be considered a secular or an ecclesiastical body, or a combination of the two. It was summarily concluded that the Hospital of San Giovanni was secular, and therefore subject to the sovereign. It thereby followed that the claims advanced by the board of governors were invalid. After some delay, the Opera Partorienti with ten beds was finally set up, and the Hospital had to foot the bill.[28]

The decision on the legal status of the hospital cleared the way for more systematic interventions by the central authority. Soon afterwards, in 1730, a 'protector' was appointed to the Hospital of San Giovanni, as shortly occurred in all charitable institutions. The protector was a high official (in this instance, the first president *pro tempore* of the Senate) who was supposed to serve as the link between the everyday running of the hospital by the board of governors, the needs of the institution, and the policies of the central government.[29] The imposition of an external authority was obviously greeted with hostility by the governors. Yet again, in 1740, an important *rappresentanza* was presented to the King in which the governors described the course conflicts had taken over several years. It included proposals for the restoration of the board's prerogatives, headed by the call for the reconsideration of the post of protector. It requested 'the First President of the Senate continue as Protector of the Hospital, providing counsel, favour and help, when the Governors and administrators so request and without interfering in the affairs and management of the Hospital'.[30] The most serious causes of the conflict date back to 1734. When faced with a grave crisis resulting in a large increase in patient admissions to the Hospital, the protector, Caissotti, imposed solutions that were at odds with the normal financial prudence of the board, leaving the Hospital deep in debt until the 1750s.[31]

Therefore, the reforms were carried out in an already highly-charged atmosphere, and represented an opportunity for further reducing the governors' authority. With the pretext of wanting to avoid straining the Hospital's finances, it was established that only a fraction of the salaries of the four physicians (whose numbers had been increased to meet the growth in teaching duties) would be paid by the Hospital itself, and the rest by the university. This seems to have had the effect of cutting down the governors' authority over the physicians and emphasising their role as teachers, as against their obligations towards the sick. Then, in 1739, the board was suddenly deprived of its traditional prerogative of selecting physicians. The central authority claimed that the physicians recently selected by the board were not up to the standards required of the post.[32] The same year it was established that the dressers would no longer be provided by the board but by the *magistrati della riforma* (the officers who governed the university),[33] and they would be chosen instead from among the surgical students at the Collegio delle Province (an institution created to promote university education via the provision of scholarships to over 200 students). The governors, in the 1740 *rappresentanza* cited above, give the impression that they were less and less in control of the management of the hospital, which was said to be slipping into chaos:

> Physicians of the hospital occasionally delegate their rounds to one another, sometimes to no one, and then send the assistant physician out on the rounds, and the chief physician comes in the evening when he can. The surgeon is deemed to have great theoretical ability but insufficient practical experience, and although it is his duty to carry out the difficult operations of removing gall stones, cleansing cataracts, suturing arteries or performing surgery on what is called the 'king's evil' [scrofula] and similar things, these duties are actually performed by former surgeons of the hospital – the Vernas, uncle and nephew. . . . The hospital is full of praise for royal provision that physicians and surgeons also be professors at the University. However, conscience requires it be reported that it is not advantageous to the Hospital because neither the physician nor the surgeon has a real dependence on it, and is harmful to the sick because they are no longer served with the punctuality and charitable feeling of before.

The very midwife of the maternity ward and school for

midwifery mentioned earlier is referred to as someone who:

> does not think of herself as depending on the Governors
> of the Hospital but on the Reform officers. She has not
> rendered service in keeping either with the rules or with
> her duty. Considerable disorder has taken place, and she
> has been absent for over three months from her post,
> having returned to her country with the intention of
> coming back the following spring. She has delegated her
> duties to another Frenchwoman, and left asking permis-
> sion only of those under whose authority she believes to
> be.

Although authority remained in the governors' hands on
paper, in practice the influence of the state officials was
greatly extended, so that the two confronted one another
inside the Hospital. Confrontations also took place at a
symbolic level, as can be seen in the episode recounted (with
a touch of irony) in the *rappresentanza*. A visitation occurs in
response to the governors' complaints that the sick were not
properly cared for by the young medical students of the
Collegio delle Province:

> Leaving aside the various acts of insolence committed,
> the First President, Protector and Head of the Reform
> came with all the Reform officials to see about the above
> mentioned inefficiencies, but did not manage to, and so
> returned a second time, with full pomp and ceremony,
> once more accompanied by all the Reform officers and,
> in addition, the Secretary of the Reform, in the light of
> which the governors argued that from then on the run-
> ning of the Hospital should fall to him, or at least the
> presiding over the governors.

We know now that what was proposed in this instance as a
possibility not without paradoxes shortly became a reality.
From the 1750s, a *magistrato della riforma* sat regularly on the
board of governors, which, by this time, no longer represented an expression of municipal power.

The reforms, it can therefore be said, did not lead to a
rationalization of the hospital's operation, but did lead to a
fairly prolonged period of confusion and poor organization

following the collapse of the traditional supervision of the medical staff's activities. The reforms were not an aspect of a conflict between 'progress' and 'backwardness', nor did they add up to a 'modernization' of the Hospital. Rather, they allowed a change of power that also occurred in other charitable institutions, not to mention the various centres of government in the city (the council, the different courts of law, and so on). The state was increasingly involved in the management of the Hospital of San Giovanni, but this did not entail any major changes in the methods of management. Inadequate provision lasted until the end of the century; 'The professors of the University do only one round a day, some go months, others years without setting foot in the Hospital. . . . The result is that the sick get inexpert and improper treatment from the two young physicians'.[34] Moreover, the innovations introduced in the financial running of the Hospital, as we have seen, turned out to be a failure. Nor was an effort made to resolve the problem of the disproportionate number of beds for incurables; on the eve of the French takeover, there were still some 218 for incurables and 232 beds for curable patients.

The shifts in the administration of charity into the hands of the state is usually in itself considered a sign of progress and rationalization. When the outcome does not meet expectations, the explanation is sought in the persistence of old forms of management, such as the continued presence of religious staff in the hospitals. My reconstruction, however, demonstrates how this shift should, in actuality, be seen as the substitution of an old elite by a new one, and as the affirmation of a new social group. In this instance, we have the state officials who concentrate power in their hands that had previously been divided up in a more complex way between different *milieux*.

It is undeniable that the appearance of a new group whose identity was now completely defined in relation to state service led a professionalization to the forms of public administration. However, it is important also to turn this perspective on its head, and observe how the rhetoric of reform and public welfare itself largely constituted a 'language' or 'discourse' that permitted or legitimized the creation of new functions and duties enlarging the scope for intervention by public administrators and the bureaucratic

117

class itself. We have seen this in the innovations introduced in the Hospital of San Giovanni, such as the Opera Partorienti, the school of midwifery, the introduction of university education to the whole hospital. These innovations can be seen as important moments in the evolution of the hospital, but they were also prongs in the attack which allowed state officials to substitute themselves for a multiplicity of different centres of power. Necessary importance should therefore be accorded to conflict as a motor of change. The clash between different groups of elites has reappeared throughout the course of this reconstruction as a crucial element in explaining developments in philanthropic practices, changes in institutional structures, and in the social composition of recipients of relief. The transformation undergone by the governing bodies of the institutions led, among other things, to a redefinition of the categories and contents of privilege. In the second half of the eighteenth century, state officials and the military progressively gained preferential access to charitable resources. In short, the establishment of state control did not entail the suppression of particularist interests in public administration, but a shift in the traditional system of protection and patronage in favour of different social groups.

Notes

1. The tendency to consider the problem of relief as the product of religious and state policies and ideologies is, above all, a feature of historiography of the 1970s, which saw a renewal of interest in the subject after a period of neglect. The findings of this research are analysed by M. Rosa in 'Chiesa, idee sui poveri e assistenza in Italia dal Cinque al Settecento', *Società e Storia*, 10 (1980). Some general syntheses on systems of poor relief in Italy come under the same heading: B. Geremek, 'Il pauperismo nell'Italia pre-industriale (sec. XIV–XVIII)', *Storia d'Italia*, vol. 5:1, *I Documenti* (Turin, 1973); B.S. Pullan, 'Poveri, mendicanti, e vagabondi (secoli XIV-XVII)', *Storia d'Italia, Annali I, Dal feudalesimo al capitalismo* (Turin, 1978); S.J. Woolf, 'La formazione del proletariato (secoli XVIII–XIX), op. cit. See also the collection of essays *Ricerche per la storia religiosa di Roma*, 3 (1979). More recently an approach that is more attentive to social dynamics is E. Grendi, 'Ideologia della carità e società indisciplinata. La costruzione del sistema assistenziale genovese', in G. Politi, M. Rosa, and F. della Peruta (eds),

Timore e carità. I poveri nell'Italia moderna (Cremona, 1982), and the number of *Quaderni Storici* edited by the same author 'Sistemi di carità. Esposti e internati nella società di Antico Regime', *Quaderni Storici*, 53 (1983). See, furthermore, the studies indicated in note 8, and the remarks by S.J. Woolf in the Introduction to his *The Poor in Western Europe in the Eighteenth and Nineteenth Centuries* (London and New York, 1986).

2. A. Scotti, 'Malati e strutture ospedaliere dall' età dei Lumi all' Unita', in F. della Peruta (ed.), *Storia d'Italia. Annali 7. Malattia e medicina* (Turin, 1984); E. Brambilla, 'La medicina nel settecento: dal monopolio dogmatico alla professione scientifica', op. cit.; P. Frascani, *Ospedale e società in età liberale* (Bologna, 1986); G. Cosmacini, *Storia della medicina e della sanità in Italia* (Bari, 1987). A different approach is developed by F. Giusberti, in the article 'La povertà e malattia. Il Sant' Orsola a Bologna dal XVII al XVIII secolo', *Annali della Fondazione Luigi Einaudi*, 13 (1979).

3. The Savoy Kingdom included after the treaty of Utrecht (1713) the territories of Piedmont, Savoy, Nice, Oneglia, Aosta, and, after 1720, Sardinia. For a classic interpretation of its political system see G. Quazza, *Le riforme in Piemonte nella prima metà del Settecento* (Modena, 1957), and more recently G. Symcox, *Victor Amadeus II. Absolutism in the Savoyard State 1675–1730* (London,1983).

4. For histories of the two hospitals, see S. Solero, *Storia dell' Ospedale Maggiore di San Giovanni Battista e della Città di Torino* (Turin, 1959); T.M. Caffaratto, *L'Ospedale Maggiore di San Giovanni Battista e della Città di Torino. Sette secoli di assistenza secoli-sanitaria* (Turin, 1984); also 'Storia dell' Ospedale Maggiore di Torino della religione e ordine dei SS. Maurizio e Lazzaro', *Annali Ospedale M. Vittoria di Torino*, XXII (1979), 7–12. During the eighteenth century the number of beds in the Hospital of S. Giovanni rose to 450 (for both curables and incurables), while the number at SS. Maurizio e Lazzaro remained at fifty to sixty.

5. These measures are mostly concentrated in the second half of the sixteenth century; T.M Caffaratto, *L'Ospedale Maggiore*, 15–16. But already, by the beginning of the seventeenth century, the city council's request that the hospital concern itself with the poor provoked the governors' protests; Archivio Comunale di Torino (henceforth ACT), *Ordinati*, 13.12.1601, 26.12.1601, 11.1.1602. The hospital, in as much as it was dependent on the municipality, carried out its duty of taking in foundlings abandoned in the city. They were then sent to the villages of the Canavese area for wet-nursing at city expense. When 10 years old, they returned to the hospital which tried to place them in apprenticeships or in service, or put up for adoption. However, with the increase in abandoned children, it became more and more difficult to find an occupation for all of them. Thus, small manufactories were organized, initially in the hospital itself, then, in the second half of the eighteenth century, on a larger scale outside the hospital.

6. As far as the Ospedale di Carità is concerned, see my article 'Conceptions of poverty and poor relief in Turin in the second half of the eighteenth century', European Institute, Florence (forthcoming). The research is based in particular on analyses of the wealth of information found in the registers of inmates kept from 1742 onwards.

7. C. Bloch, *L'assistance e L'État en France à la vieille de la Révolution, 1764–1790* (Paris, 1908); C. Jones, *Charity and Bienfaisance. The Treatment of the Poor in the Montpellier Region, 1740–1815* (Cambridge, 1982); M. Jimenez Salas, *Historia de la asistencia social en Espana en la edad moderna* (Madrid, 1958); A. Highmore, *Pietas Londiniensis* (London, 1814).

8. An important exception is the work of R. Trexler, 'Charity and defence of the urban elites in the Italian communes', in S.C. Jaher (ed.), *The Rich and the Well-born and the Powerful* (Urbana, 1973), and of G. Ricci, 'Povertà vergogna e povertà vergognosa', *Società e Storia*, 5 (1979). Worth noting is also the article by G. Muto, 'Forme e contenuti economici dell' assistenza nel Mezzogiorno moderno: il caso di Napoli', in G. Politi, M. Rosa, and F. Della Peruta (eds), *Timore e carità*. Great interest has been shown in the last few years in the study of women's institutions: L. Ciammitti, 'Fanciulle, monache, madri. Povertà femminile e previdenza a Bologne nei secoli XVI–XVIII', in *Arte e pietà. I patrimoni culturali delle opere pie* (Bologna, 1980), and 'Quanto costa essere normali. La dote nel conservatorio femminile di Santa Maria del Barracano (1630–80)', *Quaderni Storici*, 53 (1983); S. Cavallo, 'Assistenza femminile e tutela dell'onore nella Torino del XVIII secolo', *Annali della Fondazione Luigi Einaudi*, XIV (1980); L. Ferrante, 'L'onore ritrovato. Donne nella Casa del Soccorso di San Paolo a Bologna (sec. XVI–XVII)', *Quaderni Storici*, 53 (1983), D. Lombardi, 'L'ospedale dei mendicanti nella Firenze del Seicento. "Da inutile serraglio dei mendici a conservatorio e casa di forza per le donne"', *Società e Storia*, 24 (1984).

9. R. De Maio, *Società e Vita religiosa a Napoli* (Naples, 1971), 368; L. Guidi, 'Onore e status femminile negli istituti di reclusione napoletani dell' Ottocento', in *Quaderni del Dipartimento di Scienze Sociali dell' Istituto Universitario Orientale di Napoli*, 2 (1988); S. Cavallo, 'Assistenza femminile'.

10. For an interpretation of women's institutions as a product of the cultural climate of the Counter Reformation see B. Pullan, *Rich and Poor in Renaissance Venice: The Social Institutions of a Catholic State to 1620* (Oxford, 1971), 385–94, and 'The old Catholicism, the new Catholicism and the poor', in G. Politi, M. Rosa, and F. della Peruta (eds), *Timore e carità*, 16–17. For explanations of the widespread relief to the shamefaced poor see G. Ricci, 'Povertà, vergogna', 328–9.

11. Archivio Storico San Paolo, *Ordinati*, vol. III, n. 57, 21.2.1734.

12. Archivio Storico San Paolo, *Repertorio dei lasciti*, vol. 160–163.

13. Archivio Ospedale San Giovanni (henceforth AOSG), *Ordinati*, 26.6.1667, 9.3.1668.

14. The endowments of beds for incurables have been reconstructed using various sources: the fund *Letti Incurabili* (AOSG, Categoria 10, Classe 3, vols 1–7) has in fact turned out to be incomplete. Further documentation was obtained therefore from the fund *Eredità Legati* (AOSG, Categoria 4, Classe 1, vols 1–69), and from the *Ordinati* of the hospital from 1668 onwards. The beds were put up either by donations of living donors, or left in wills; in this second case a rather long time possibly passed from the disposition to the actual foundation. Note that the dates given here (including those that appear in Table 4.1) refer to the disposition; that is the official act which the benefactor provided for the immediate or future foundation.

15. AOSG, *Ordinati*, 10.4.1713, 10.12.1716, 6.12.1723, 30.12.1724.

16. The formula for the endowment of beds stipulated that incurables be expelled if they failed to show respect for hospital officials or caused disorder. There are actually some cases of expulsion documented.

17. Archivio di Stato di Torino, *Luoghi Pii di qua dai Monti*, m.19, fasc.7, 'Sentimenti sugeriti dal principe di Francavilla e dal Padre Perardo. . . circa il modo di promuovere il sovenimento dei poveri', 1734.

18. AOSG, *Ordinati*, 21.5.1744.

19. AOSG, *Ordinati*, 21.1.1754, 27.5.1775. In January 1760, for example, since money was needed for the completion of the hospital buildings, the governors put twenty-three entitlements for the nomination of beds for incurables up for sale at 3,000 lire each following their reversion to the hospital on the death of the testators' descendents. Some twenty-one were sold within a year. AOSG, *Ordinati*, 16.1.1760.

20. AOSG, *Ordinati*, 20.4.1780.

21. See M. Vovelle, *Piété baroque et déchristianisation en Provence au XVIIIe siècle* (Paris, 1978).

22. G. Prato, *Problemi monetari e bancari nei secoli XVII e XVIII* (Torino, 1916).

23. OSG, Cat. 10, Cl. 3, vol. 2.

24. 'Il modo et governo de la Congregatione de poveri in l'hospitale di San Giovanni', 1.5.1541, published in T.M. Caffaratto, *L'Ospedale Maggiore*, 195, *passim*.

25. All information about the extent and increase of the medical staff, the careers of physicians and surgeons, was obtained through examination of the hospital *Ordinati*. Some biographical information relative to physicians and surgeons can be found in G.G. Bonino, *Biografia medica piemontese*, 2 vols (Turin, 1925).

26. F.A. Duboin, *Raccolta per ordine di materie delle leggi . . . emanate*

negli stati di terraferma fino all'8 dicembre 1798 dai sovrani della real casa di Savoia (Turin, 1818–68), T. XIV, Capo IV, 'Dell'insegnamento della medicina', 643–49; Cap V, 'Dell' insegnamento della Chirurgia', 655–66; Articolo IV, 723; Articolo V, 733. T. Vallauri, *Storia delle Università degli Studi del Piemonte*, 3 vols (Turin, 1816). D. Balani, D. Carpanetto, and F. Turletti, 'La popolazione studentesca dell' Università di Torino nel Settecento', *Bollettino Storico Bibliografico Subalpino*, LXXVI (1978).

27. J.J. Bylebyl, 'Commentary', in J.H. Stevenson, *A Celebration of Medical History* (Baltimore and London, 1982). For a re-evaluation of the hospital's role as a place for medical practice, research, and training in other areas of Europe besides Paris in the eighteenth century, see O. Keel, 'The politics of health and the institutionalisation of clinical practices in Europe in the second half of the eighteenth century', in W.F. Bynum and R. Porter (eds), *William Hunter and the Eighteenth-Century Medical World* (Cambridge, 1985). For reforms in Tuscany and Lombardy during 1770s and 1780s see A. Scotti, 'Malati e strutture ospedaliere', 250 *passim*; G. Cosmacini, *Storia della medicina*, 234 *passim*.

28. The conflict over the foundation of the Opera Partorienti can be followed in the minute books (*Ordinati*) from the board of governors meetings.

29. F.A. Duboin, *Raccolta*, T. XII, 647, 'Regie Patenti di nomina del Primo Presidente del Senato di Piemonte, con autorità di vegliare al buon governo dell'ospedale di San Giovanni in Torino', 10.8.1730.

30. ACT, *Ospedale di San Giovanni*, N.666, 'Rappresentanza del venerando spedale maggiore di San Giovanni Battista e della città di Torino', 1740.

31. Caissotti ordered that the hospital, already overflowing with patients, should try to accept all the sick who asked to be admitted, by creating new beds, transforming areas used for other purposes into patient-care areas, and increasing the number of physicians and nurses. To this purpose all of the hospital income had to be used (including the reserve that the board of governors usually kept intact) and the hospital had to resort to loans for further financing (AOSG, *Ordinati*, 29.6.1734).

32. AOSG, *Ordinati*, 9.8.1739.

33. AOSG, *Ordinati*, 2.8.1739.

34. T.M. Caffaratto, *L'Ospedale Maggiore*, 143, 'Relazione anonima', toward the end of the century.

5

Politics and the London Royal Hospitals, 1683 – 92[1]

Craig Rose

Between 1546 and 1552 Henry VIII and Edward VI established, on the site of dissolved monastic foundations, the five London royal hospitals: St Bartholomew's, St Thomas's, Christ's, Bridewell, and Bethlem. Although they were the largest and wealthiest charitable institutions in early modern London, their early history has been virtually ignored by professional historians. Those interested in the hospitals are thus still largely dependent on the staid and reverential institutional histories written in the first decades of this century.[2] The lack of interest of social and medical historians in the royal hospitals is understandable; prior to the late eighteenth century the hospital records contain only minimal information on medical practices and the conditions of patients and inmates. The neglect of political historians is less excusable. The royal hospitals were important civic institutions, and were bound to be affected by major crises in civic politics. One such crisis in London politics broke out in the last years of the reign of Charles II.

The early 1680s witnessed a vicious struggle for power in London between the emergent Whig and Tory parties. When victory in that battle had gone to the Tory supporters of Charles II, the King and his government launched a systematic effort to drive the Whigs from public life. With their extensive property-holdings and substantial revenues, the royal hospitals, especially Whig-dominated St Thomas's, soon drew the attention of the authorities. In 1683 the Crown intervened in the administration of the hospitals, and purged those governors and staff members who supported the Whigs. After 1683 the Stuart monarchy and the political parties

123

experienced many vicissitudes, which were also reflected in the affairs of the hospitals. In this essay, I shall explain how and why these philanthropic institutions were drawn into the bitter conflict between Whigs and Tories.

The administration of the Royal Hospitals

The royal hospitals established in the mid-Tudor period were apparently London's response to the municipal relief institutions which had recently been opened at Lyon and Geneva.[3] The hospitals were each allocated specific tasks: St Bartholomew's, West Smithfield, and St Thomas's, Southwark, the two greatest of the medieval hospitals, were to provide relief for the sick poor; Christ's Hospital was to cater for the orphaned children of poor City freemen; Bridewell, a former royal palace, was converted into a correction centre for vagrants; and Bethlem retained its pre-Reformation role as a lunatic asylum.

Although the hospitals were royal foundations, their administration was placed in the hands of the Corporation of London. At first the hospitals were closely supervised by the City authorities. An Act of Common Council of 1557 required yearly joint elections of governors, under aldermanic supervision, at Christ's Hospital on St Matthew's Day (21 September); in the same year a joint rule book was issued.[4] In practice, apart from Bridewell and Bethlem which shared a single administration, the hospitals soon went their separate ways. Aldermanic supervision of the governors had lapsed by 1615, and though the St Matthew's Day Court continued, its function had become purely ceremonial.[5] By the early years of the seventeenth century, though they continued to receive certain customary revenues from the City, the hospitals had become virtually independent corporations.

Each hospital was ruled by a court of governors, which elected its own members, appointed hospital staff, and chose a new president from the ranks of the City aldermen upon the death or retirement of the incumbent. The president himself had sole power to convene meetings of the General Court of Governors, and a dominant president could have a decisive influence on its proceedings. The General Court met relatively infrequently, and day-to-day administration was in the hands of a committee of governors centred on the treasurer. Its decisions were provisional, and required the approval of the General Court for ratification.

Most of the governors' time was taken up with mundane administrative matters: renewing leases on hospital property; entering into contracts with tradesmen; and ensuring the maintenance of the hospital buildings. They do not appear to have supervised the welfare of patients and inmates closely. The relief activities of the hospitals, however, were considerable. In 1677–8 St Bartholomew's Hospital provided treatment for 1,967 patients, and its sister hospital of St Thomas's for 2,080. Both hospitals also gave 'money and other necessaries' to patients on their discharge. Christ's Hospital was providing for the education and upkeep of 663 poor children in 1684.[6] To finance these activities, the hospitals relied upon their own large, independent revenues, derived primarily from endowed property. Thus by the 1680s the annual revenues of St Bartholomew's and Christ's Hospitals both exceeded £7,000, while those of St Thomas's totalled more than £4,000.[7]

The independence of the hospitals, though, was largely illusory. Aldermanic control of the hospitals, embodied in the original royal grant of the institutions to the City, had lapsed but had never been legally revoked. Even more importantly, as royal foundations the hospitals were ultimately subject to the authority of the Crown. Indeed, in the letters patent of 1552, by which he granted Christ's, Bridewell, and Bethlem to the City, Edward VI specifically reserved the right for his 'Heirs and Successors' to appoint commissioners, if they saw fit, 'to visit the Hospitalls . . . and to doe and execute' all matters relating to their management.[8] The hospitals' double vulnerability to outside intervention was to be graphically exposed during the political crisis that racked the nation after the Popish Plot revelations of 1678.

Sir John Lawrence and St Thomas's Hospital

From 1679 to 1681 the Earl of Shaftesbury's exploitation of the mass hysteria generated by the Plot seemed to have the throne of the Stuarts once again teetering on the edge of collapse. In three successive general elections Shaftesbury's

Whigs had gained victory, but they had not achieved power; by skilful use of his prerogative rights of proroguing and dissolving Parliament, Charles II had thwarted the Whigs' efforts to exclude his Catholic brother and heir, James, Duke of York, from the succession to the throne.[9] By 1681 the Crown's steadily improving financial position enabled Charles to rule without Parliament, and he launched a counter-attack against his enemies. In the last four years of his reign, the so-called Tory reaction, the King co-operated with his Tory supporters in systematically driving the Whigs from public life. The Whig leaders were struck down one by one. Protestant dissenters, the strongest supporters of the Whigs, were persecuted with relentless zeal by Tory justices.[10] The most ambitious aspect of the royal offensive was a wholesale attack on parliamentary corporations. Through the issue of writs of *quo warranto*, corporation charters were forfeited and remodelled by the Crown to bring them under its control.

The dominance of London in the nation's affairs naturally made it a focal point in the Crown-Tory campaign. In the capital the battle between Whigs and Tories was particularly fierce, and from 1682 began to run decisively in favour of the Tories.[11] Victory in a bitterly contested shrieval election brought the Tories control of the City's law courts. The charters of several City livery companies were forfeited, and hundreds of Whig liverymen were purged, thus disqualifying them from voting in mayoral, shrieval, and parliamentary elections. Most dramatically of all, a *quo warranto* was issued against the Corporation of London itself. As a result, in October 1683 the City's charter was forfeited, the Corporation of London dissolved, and the City was placed directly under the control of royal commissioners.[12] As we shall soon see, one of the tasks entrusted to the commissioners was to purge the royal hospitals of all parties disaffected to the government.

The first sign that the Tory reaction in London would extend as far as the hospitals had come in 1682. On 9 February the Tory-controlled Court of Aldermen issued an order that the hospitals should appoint no further governors without the Court's approval, thus reasserting a power that had lapsed for over sixty years. Two weeks later an aldermanic committee was established to investigate the hospitals' administration.[13]

Within a few days these sudden efforts of the aldermen to reassert their ancient authority over the hospitals were overtaken by a more serious development. On 27 February the General Court of Governors of St. Thomas's Hospital received the stunning news that a Royal Commission of Visitation had been established to examine the affairs of that hospital.[14] This initial royal intervention does not appear to have progressed very far, and no action was taken against St Thomas's. Nevertheless the events of spring 1682 had shown that both the Court of Aldermen and the Crown were concerned about the hospitals, and that St Thomas's was the primary object of their concern.

Why had St Thomas's attracted such undesired attention? The answer lies primarily in government suspicion of Alderman Sir John Lawrence, president of St Thomas's since 1668. A wealthy City merchant, Lawrence was a man of strength and courage; Lord Mayor during the Great Plague of 1665, he had been one of the few to stay at his post throughout that terrible episode.[15] He was also an inveterate and tactless opponent of Charles II's regime; as early as 1672 a government informant was warning of the 'imperious and insolent behaviour' of the 'ill minded' Lawrence, and of his attempts to fan hostility to the government in the City.[16] During the exclusion crisis Lawrence was a senior figure among the City Whigs, and in 1681 he had been foreman of Shaftesbury's *ignoramus* jury.[17]

According to complaints made to the King by some disgruntled Southwark Tories, Lawrence's Whiggery was having a major impact on the administration of St Thomas's. The Tories claimed that Sir John and the hospital's Nonconformist treasurer, James Hayes, had appropriated to themselves the power to appoint governors. Consequently 'a very great Majority [of the Court]' were said to be 'persons avowedly disaffected to the Government established'.[18] This appears to be something of an exaggeration. I have identified 102 of the governors of St Thomas's in 1683, although the total number was probably closer to 130.[19] Of these 102 I have labelled forty as Tories and forty-two as Whigs, with at least ten of the latter being dissenters.[20] However, holding the key positions of president and treasurer, the Whigs certainly exercised a dominant influence on the hospital's affairs. Their power was clearly reflected in the composition of the hospital's staff and appointees. Although the rector of the parish of St Thomas was 'a person of inflexible loyalty' to the government, the remaining hospital appointees, from the chaplain, William Hughes, and the physician, Richard Torlesse, 'down to the porters', were all said to be persons of 'factious principles'.[21]

This was most obviously so in the case of the chaplain, or hospitaller, William Hughes. During the Civil War Hughes had been a chaplain in the parliamentary army, and as a reward had gained the rich living of Hinton in Berkshire.[22] In 1651 he had delivered a sermon in which he argued that the age of the fifth monarchy was dawning, and that the regicide was 'not so uncouth as some do render it', having 'cured the wound' of monarchy, that persecutor of the saints.[23] When that 'wound' was reopened in 1660 Hughes was ejected from Hinton, and for some time thereafter was patronized by Lord Wharton, the leading Presbyterian peer.[24] By 1680, the year in which he was appointed chaplain of St Thomas's, Hughes was edging towards conformity.[25] But it was not until three years after his appointment to St Thomas's that he conformed to the Church of England and was ordained.[26] It is clear, though, that Hughes was an unenthusiastic Anglican, for in July 1683 the King ordered the Bishop of Winchester to investigate complaints 'of the great disorderliness in the Church service as now performed in St Thomas' Hospital, Southwark, to the great discouragement of loyal and conformable subjects'.[27] A later report gave a colourful if somewhat jaundiced account of Hughes's unease with the Church of England: 'the Form of Prayer made him puke, he sweat at the Litany . . . and he still hates every thing in the Church but its Preferments'.[28]

The maintenance of a Nonconformist chaplain is the most blatant sign of the political and religious sympathies of the dominant group of governors led by Sir John Lawrence. More important was the Whigs' exploitation of the hospital's extensive properties and revenues as a means of political influence and patronage in Southwark. St Thomas's owned 170 rents in the borough, 110 of these in the parish of St Thomas itself, where virtually all property was in the hospital's hands.[29] The parliamentary franchise in Southwark was vested in all householders not in receipt of alms,[30] so the hospital's property gave it a major influence over a considerable number of votes. According to the Tories the governors had fully exploited this influence on behalf of the Whig candidates in the hard-fought Southwark election of 1681, 'showing favour or using Rigor in renewing leases' to tenants, 'accordingly as they act agreeably or contrary to their dictates'.[31]

Another major source of local patronage for the governors was the disbursement of the hospital's revenues. In 1681–2 St Thomas's income amounted to £4,147, derived primarily from its rentals. Disbursements in that year totalled almost £4,000, of which £2,130 were expended on tradesmen's contracts, mainly for food and other supplies for the patients.[32] With such spending power, the governors could exercise a major influence over local traders. Indeed in October 1683 a government informant had warned secretary of state Jenkins that the disposal of hospital revenues was of great importance to London tradesmen, and that where a hospital's 'officers are factious, the revenues are disposed of to their own party to the discouragement of loyal citizens'. He concluded, 'I need not mention St Thomas, where the whole revenue is and has been distributed amongst the enemies of the government.'[33]

By 1683 Tory fears about St Thomas's role in fomenting and sustaining Whiggery in Southwark had reached fever-pitch. In January the Southwark grand jury urged local justices 'to increase the number and strengthen the interest' of the loyal party in the borough, who were 'labouring more particularly under the grievance, that persons notoriously disaffected are become the majority of governors of an hospital of royal foundation among them and so the disposers of all offices relating thereto and the managers of a large revenue belonging thereto'.[34] That summer it was reported that the loyalty of Southwark was 'preserved only by the care of a few honest and active men'; among the measures recommended to curb opposition was the visitation of St Thomas's.[35]

The Commission for Hospitals 1683–8

The opportunity to take action against St Thomas's and disaffected elements in the other hospitals came in October

1683, when the dissolution of the Corporation of London and the purge of the Whig minority on the aldermanic bench marked the complete defeat of the City Whigs. On 15 October it was urged upon secretary Jenkins that 'In the regulation his Majesty is now about concerning the City, great care should be taken in the government of the hospitals.'[36] On 20 October, Lord Mayor Sir William Pritchard instructed the Common Sergeant of London to search the poll books, in order to discover how the hospital staff had voted in elections; the previous day the Common Sergeant and the Recorder had 'settled a commission for the government of the hospitals'.[37] A royal warrant was issued on 23 October, appointing the Commission, whose membership was identical with that of the Commission to rule the City – the Crown and the City law officers, the Lord Mayor, and the purged Court of Aldermen.[38] It appears that no independent action was thought necessary against the hospital charters, since their fate was deemed to be bound up with that of the demised Corporation of London.

The first meeting of the Commission for Hospitals took place on 10 November, when the royal hospitals were purged of the Whigs among their governors and staffs, and their replacements appointed.[39] Heeding the informant's recommendations on the revenues, the Commissioners ordered that the hospitals should only employ such tradesmen 'as are truely Loyall and well affected to the government'. They also required the clerks of the hospitals to furnish lists of their tenants. This indicates that the commissioners were fully aware of the political significance of the hospitals' property, and that they perhaps intended to cow disaffected tenants by threat of eviction. Since 1682 the Tory justices in the London area had been fighting an economic war against the dissenters, linking the licensing of innholders and the payment of poor relief to church attendance; the commissioners' orders on tradesmen and tenants should be seen in this context.[40]

The impact of the Commission varied greatly from hospital to hospital. Not surprisingly St Thomas's, which had prompted the intervention in the first place, was the worst hit. The president, Sir John Lawrence, was replaced by Sir William Hooker, a Tory alderman, while the treasurer was also displaced. The total number of governors ejected is unknown, but was probably well over forty.[41] To replace them the commissioners appointed a large number of new governors.[42] Virtually the entire staff was ejected. Out went William Hughes, the chaplain; Dr. Richard Torlesse, the physician; Thomas Hollyer, one of the surgeons; the steward; the clerk and his rent-gatherer, the porters, and the beadle.[43] In August 1684 the hospital's remodelled Court of Governors was also to dismiss six of the nursing staff, including three sisters, for 'incorrigible ill behaviour' and 'non complyance with the rules and orders of this House'.[44]

For Whigs and Nonconformists in Southwark, the loss of hospital contracts and the threat of eviction must have been a severe blow. As early as 27 October the Surrey justices, three of whom were Tory governors of St Thomas's, reported that vigorous prosecution of the penal laws had forced many Southwark dissenters to 'leave their trades and habitations'. 'This prosecution being continued', they wrote, 'and our Hospital Regulated (a matter of so great Consequence in the whole affair, that we cannot omit to mention it whenever we speak of Southwark), we shall shortly be able to give you as good an account of this borough as you can wish'.[45]

Were there also attempts to bar dissenters from entering the hospital as patients? From 1689 to 1690 John Turner, the chaplain appointed by the commissioners in 1683, fought a desperate battle to prevent his dismissal by the resurgent Whigs.[46] During this struggle he twice expressed his hostility to discrimination against patients on the grounds of religion, which at least suggests that such an accusation had been made.[47] However, in the absence of any firmer evidence it seems best to deliver a 'not proven' verdict on this issue.

Of the other hospitals, Christ's was the next worst affected by the rule of the commissioners. The president, Sir John Frederick, was a Whig alderman, while the treasurer and several of the governors were described as 'old Cromwellists'.[48] All were dismissed. Three new governors were appointed by the commissioners, and on 11 December the remodelled Christ's General Court appointed nineteen more. Only two of the hospital's employees were dismissed – the girls' school mistress, and the master of a school administered by the hospital at Ware in Hertfordshire.[49] At Bridewell, where Sir William Turner, a devout churchman, was president, the only major casualty was the hospital's treasurer.[50]

The hospital least touched by these events was St Bartholomew's. During the Civil War St Bartholomew's apparently acquired a reputation as a stronghold of Anglican royalism, and in the early 1680s its Court of Governors was composed almost entirely of Tories.[51] In November 1682 the governors anticipated a later measure by the commissioners, when they ordered 'That noe person or persons whatsoever that shall dissent from the Church of England or are disaffected with the Government as is now established by law shall serve this Hospitall with any Comoditties'.[52] With such fervent loyalty among the governors there was little for the commissioners to do, and hospital affairs after November 1683 were conducted much as before.

In February 1685 the Catholic James II succeeded to the throne. For the first year of his reign the Anglican *status quo* was maintained, but by early 1686 the King had made it clear that he wished to introduce toleration and civil equality for his co-religionists. When his Tory allies refused to accept such a policy, James began to co-operate with his erstwhile enemies, the Whigs and Nonconformists. Thus from late 1686 it was the Tories who were to find themselves under attack from royal power.

The first hospital to feel the effects of King James's policies was staunchly Tory St Bartholomew's, whose governors now faced a far greater degree of intervention in their affairs. Although power to appoint governors and staff lay with the commissioners, it is clear that prior to 1687 they only confirmed selections presented to them by the Court of Governors. However, in March 1687 the commissioners appointed an officer without reference to the governors.[53] Three months later the governors were informed that it was 'his Majesties pleasure' that his personal druggist, a certain Staines, be appointed the hospital druggist. The governors were disgruntled; though they 'frankly complied' with the King's command, they warned Staines to 'serve the house with as good drugs and att as reasonable price as any other person, hath, or will do'.[54] In November, when the King appointed Timothy Sutton assistant surgeon, the governors' unhappiness was even more evident. Most unusually, they pointedly warned Sutton 'to be carefull in the Busienesse that shalbe assigned him'.[55]

The governors could do little to oppose the King's orders, but they responded to his religious policies by reasserting St Bartholomew's traditional Anglicanism. In April 1686, when the vicar of the hospital parish of St Bartholomew the Less asked the governors to provide a new surplice, he was told to go to the churchwardens; a year later a surplice was 'appointed to be provided at the charge of this house'.[56] In October 1685 the parishioners of Christ Church, Newgate Street, the presentation to which lay with the hospital, asked the governors to contribute to the pewing of the church, only to receive the brusque reply that 'it did not concerne this Hospitall neither was the house in a condition to answer this request'.[57] In June 1687, shortly after James had officially granted toleration to Catholics and dissenters, the governors ordered the construction of a new altar for Christ Church at the cost of £100 to the hospital.[58] This reassertion of Anglican values was also reflected in the governors' decision in January 1688 to introduce compulsory daily prayers for the patients.[59]

By that time the King had further intervened in the affairs of the royal hospitals. In October 1687 James removed the recalcitrant Tories from the Court of Alderman.[60] Among these were the presidents of Bridewell, Christ's, and St Bartholomew's. They were now dismissed from their presidencies by the hospital commissioners, and replaced by supporters of the King.[61] The presidents were the sole victims of the purge, for there were no mass removals of governors and staff as in 1683. However, at Christ's Hospital some of the Whig governors ejected in 1683 had been restored in March 1687, and several more were reappointed a year later.[62] At St Thomas's some of the governors removed in 1683 also appear to have been restored early in 1688.[63]

The struggle for St Thomas's 1689–92

If the King had plans for a more ambitious remodelling of the hospitals' administration, then these, like his far grander designs, were swept away by the Glorious Revolution of November 1688. A month earlier, in a forlorn effort to conciliate his opponents, James had already restored the City of London's charter, thus re-establishing the Corporation and, *inter alia*, dissolving the Commission for Hospitals.[64] On 6 November the Court of Aldermen, now restored of its members purged by King Charles in 1683 and King James in 1687, set up a committee to investigate the appointment of the hospital presidents. The governors of Christ's, Bridewell, and St Bartholomew's did not await the outcome of the committee's deliberations, and swiftly restored the Tory presidents deposed in 1687.[65]

Events at St Thomas's Hospital were far more complicated. The president, Sir William Hooker, had been the only hospital president to escape the anti-Tory purge of 1687. But he now faced the challenge of Sir John Lawrence, the Whig president deposed in 1683. The Court of Governors was still composed mostly of those appointed by the commissioners in 1683. They were likely to resist fiercely the restoration of Lawrence, for if Hooker were not the rightful president then they could hardly be the rightful governors. For his part, Lawrence could rely on the support of the surviving Whig governors ejected with him in 1683 in any attempt to overthrow the work of the commissioners. A clash was inevitable.

Lawrence forced the issue by summoning a General Court, which he hoped would recognize him as president. The Court met on 10 January 1689, and was attended both by those governors ejected by the commissioners in 1683 and those that had been appointed to replace them. Immediately 'reflections and hott debate did arise', the rival groups presumably questioning each other's legality.[66] A later report alleged that the Commission governors made 'a very great disturbance', and 'would not suffer any settlement to be made'.[67] As well as refusing to accept Sir John Lawrence as president, it would appear that the Commission governors were determined to prevent the restoration of the hospital staff deposed in 1683.

On 14 January Sir William Hooker, who had avoided the meeting thanks to a strategically timed cold, wrote a letter to the aldermanic bench outlining his position on these events.[68] He regretted the altercations between the rival groups of governors, 'it being not the way to heale a Nation'. However, Hooker insisted that Sir John Lawrence could only be restored by a direct order from the aldermen. His only personal desire was that the Court of Aldermen 'take such a measure and way of settling this businesse, as that it may take away all animosities'. To this end Hooker was willing to give up the presidency. But this was only on the proviso that Lawrence 'will not insist upon any matter whereby others may suffer'; by this he meant any attempt to eject the staff appointed by the commissioners in 1683.

There was never any direct order restoring Lawrence as president, but the Court of Aldermen seem to have accepted him as such. Sir John's initial aim was to restore the hospital staff dismissed in 1683. Unable to call a General Court of Governors because of the presence of the Commission governors, Lawrence decided to work through the aldermanic bench where the Whigs were gaining the ascendancy. On 24 January the aldermen ordered the reinstatement of all ejected officers, probably on the grounds that they were legally restored by virtue of the restitution of the City charter.[69] Some of the existing hospital staff who were to be displaced by the order resisted the restoration of the former officers. This resistance was led by John Turner, who had been appointed hospital chaplain by the commissioners in 1683. In the course of 1689 he launched into a series of unavailing appeals to the aldermen to revoke their January order.[70] Finally, in the early summer of 1690 he joined forces with Dr William Briggs, the recently deposed hospital physician, in a petition to King William and Queen Mary. Their petition was referred to Lord Chief Justice Holt who settled matters by judging against Turner and Briggs in December 1690.[71]

By 1690, thanks to the Court of Aldermen, St Thomas's had been cleared of the officers appointed by the commissioners in November 1683, and those purged at that time had been restored. However, Sir John Lawrence and his supporters among the governors had not fully regained control of the hospital and its patronage. The governors appointed by the commissioners were still in the majority, and it was effectively impossible for the president to call a General Court. During this period the hospital was administered by the Grand Committee, the body of governors which normally ran affairs between Courts. Composed of governors from the rival groups, the Committee had kept St Thomas's functioning, but no binding decisions could be made without the approval of a General Court.[72] It was thus imperative for Lawrence to remove the Commission governors if he were to regain control of the hospital and its patronage.

The first moves were made in the summer of 1690. On 1 July Lawrence gained the approval of the aldermen for the appointment of fifty-nine new governors.[73] I have identified the probable political affiliation of thirty of these men: one was a Tory; two were Tories by 1700, but were political waverers in 1690; twenty-seven were Whigs.[74] Among these twenty-seven were many of the leading names of London Whiggery. Eleven of them were aldermen, virtually the entire Whig component of the aldermanic bench. Ten of the twenty-seven had had action taken against them during Monmouth's rebellion.[75] No fewer than fourteen of the twenty-five men identified by G.S. De Krey as the leaders of the London Whigs in 1690 can be found among these twenty-seven governors.[76] On the basis of such evidence there can be little doubt that most of the twenty-nine new governors whose political allegiance has proved unidentifiable were Whig in their sympathies.

His support among the governors powerfully reinforced, Lawrence was ready to take direct action against the Commission governors. The obvious method was to work through the Court of Aldermen, controlled by the Whigs since 1689.[77] Sir John had already exploited the ancient aldermanic power over the hospitals in gaining the removal of the Commission-appointed staff and the appointment of the new Whig governors; now he brought the issue of the Commission governors before the aldermen.[78] It was claimed that since January 1689 the business of the hospital had been obstructed by the Commission governors, and that the president would be unable to hold court 'until those Commission Governors were many of them laid aside'. Their original appointment had been illegal, for many were said to be 'not free of the City'. Moreover they were politically obnoxious, 'severall of them being actors in Cheife for the turning out of the ancient worthy Citizens that were Governors before the avoydance of the Charter'. In fact they had been 'the only forward men to have the Charter delivered up to the then King', and others were 'knowne to be profest Papists'. In addition the Commission governors were alleged to be indisposed to charity, being men of 'very mean estates and of a covetous mind'. It was therefore requested that the aldermen depose the Commission governors, and that in future only 'those that were Governors before the Judgement in the Quo warranto And those approved by the Court of Aldermen in July last 1690' be summoned to attend hospital courts.

On 23 October a committee of nine aldermen was established to investigate not only the St Thomas's controversy, but also the method of appointing the governors of the 'severall hospitals'. Seven of its members were governors of St Thomas's Hospital; two were Tories who had been governors since the 1670s, while five were Whigs appointed in July 1690. This left two outsiders, a Whig and a Tory, who were immediately made governors by Lawrence in an obvious bid for their support.[79]

The extension of the committee's terms of reference to the other hospitals raised the suspicions of the governors of Tory St Bartholomew's. They seem to have feared, with some justification, that it was a Whig attempt to purge all the hospitals of large numbers of Tory governors. Throughout 1691 Alderman Sir William Pritchard, president of St Bartholomew's, procrastinated in the face of repeated aldermanic commands that the hospital deliver to the committee its charter and a list of its governors. In September a compromise was at last reached; the names of the governors would be presented to the Lord Mayor, but only within the framework of the traditional and purely ceremonial St Matthew's Day Joint-Court at Christ's Hospital. Little wonder that Pritchard was thanked by the governors of St Bartholomew's for successfully 'asserting the Rights of this Hospitall'.[80]

The aldermanic committee itself was divided over the issue of the St Thomas's Commission governors. On 8 January 1691 Sir John Lawrence was informed 'that the Committee of Aldermen had a meeting last night wherein they much debated the business of our Governors but could com to no issue'. Lawrence was urged to attend the committee, for 'with your Assistance it would be carried to lay asid the Commission Governors'.[81] It appears likely that the Tory minority on the Committee was putting up a stiff defence of the Commission governors, or that some of the more moderate Whigs were wavering. It was not until 10 March that the committee reached its verdict, declaring the appointment of the Commission governors to be illegal. But the report was signed by only five of the committee's nine members, all of them Whigs.[82]

Armed with the aldermanic decision against the Commission governors, Sir John Lawrence called a General Court of St Thomas's Hospital, summoning only those governors appointed prior to the *quo warranto* or since July 1690. The Court met on 27 March 1691, the first since September 1687, and, in the opinion of Sir John and his supporters, the first legal Court since June 1683. A committee was immediately established to investigate fully the hospital's administration in the intervening eight years, but its primary purpose was to consider how many of the Commission governors 'are fitt, and propper, to be continued governors'.[83] At the next General Court on 26 May the committee presented its report, 'which being read and debated upon after some amendments was approved'. Only forty-three of the 137 Commission governors were to be retained, and few of these were to play an active part in hospital administration.[84] Lawrence and the Whigs had regained control of St Thomas's.

In only one area at St Thomas's had the events of 1683 to 1688 not yet been overturned. Three of the hospital's four surgeons had been appointed during the rule of the commissioners, although not in the original intervention of October/ November 1683.[85] It seems that as they had not been appointed directly upon the forfeiture of the City's charter, it had not been possible to remove them in 1689 upon the charter's restitution. The fourth surgeon, John Browne, had in fact been appointed by the governors in June 1683, prior to the *quo warranto*. But his appointment had been due to strong royal pressure at a time when the governors were hardly in a position to resist.[86]

In May 1691 a committee of governors reported that there were 'great animosities between the Chirugeons', and that all four were guilty of a 'breach of orders and neglect of their duty to the great prejudice of the patients'.[87] There may well have been some validity in these charges; in October 1689 the Grand Committee had suspended Browne for performing 'considerable operacons' without the approval of the physician and the other surgeons,[88] while it is possible that the surgeons were quarrelling over seniority.[89] However, the issue was complicated by the political considerations. The governors alleged that the 'cheife cause' of the surgeons' misconduct was

> the methods by which they came into their places, every one of them haveing been chosen or placed either with regard to Recomendatory Letters [as in Browne's case] or by Mandamus as in the time when Governed by Commissioners, which has made some of them say often That they were not chose by the Governors and therefore were not to obey them.[90]

On 7 July the General Court decided that the surgeons' reported misbehaviour was 'a sufficient ground for the Court to proceed to a new Election of surgeons'. Fearing the worst, John Browne then appeared, and pleaded the court's favour as 'hee was chose at a General Court'. The governors, though, were set on their course; Browne and his three colleagues were summarily dismissed.[91] Sir John Lawrence and his governors must now have fondly believed that they had finally cleansed the hospital's Augean Stables: they were soon to be proved sadly mistaken.

John Browne had been Charles II's surgeon-in-ordinary, and was a passionate high Anglican.[92] In 1684 he had written *Charisma Basilicon*, a major book on touching for the king's evil, in which ceremony he played a leading part. After the Revolution he had managed to retain royal favour, and had been appointed William III's surgeon. He was not the sort of man to take dismissal lightly. Thus, within days of their dismissal, Browne and his three colleagues had petitioned the Privy Council to overturn the governors' actions.[93] The surgeons claimed that they had been ejected 'for no other reason than that they came in by Mandates'. Some of the governors, they alleged, had 'been willing to introduce their own friends', and 'formed parties', an allusion to the appointments of July 1690. Nearly 100 rightful governors had not been summoned to the court at which the surgeons had been dismissed, a reference to the deposition of the Commission governors. Even so, they claimed, some of the governors had protested against the court's proceedings, a fascinating glimpse of possible conflict between the Whig and the few remaining Tory governors. Finally the surgeons alleged that their replacements were inexperienced, and totally unqualified for their places.

The surgeons' petition was considered by the Privy Council on 17 July. At a meeting attended by only Queen Mary and Lord President Carmarthen, it was decided to summon the governors to explain their actions at the next meeting of the Council.[94] A week later, at a much fuller meeting attended by the King, the governors presented their defence. It failed to impress the Privy Council, which decided to establish a Commission of Visitation to investigate the affair.[95] Two factors probably account for the Council's decision. In the first place St Thomas's was packed with soldiers and seamen wounded during the war with France[96]; the surgeons made great play of their services to these men, and such a dramatic turnover in the surgical staff was bound to alarm the King and the Council. This was especially so if the surgeons had been dismissed on political rather than medical grounds, and this leads naturally to the second aspect of the Council's reasoning. Since 1689 King William had become increasingly suspicious of the partisanship and radicalism of his London Whig allies, viewing their vengeful attacks on the Tories as an obstruction to the efficient prosecution of the French war. In consequence the King had turned to the Tories, still further alienating the Whigs, who now had a sense of betrayal added to their other grievances.[97] As we have seen, many of London's leading Whigs were governors of St Thomas's Hospital; the Privy Council may have interpreted the dismissal of the surgeons as a further illustration of the irresponsible partisanship of the City Whigs, not to mention a breach of the spirit of the May 1690 Act for reversing the *quo warranto*.[98]

On 18 August a warrant was issued, establishing a Royal Commission to investigate all hospitals of royal foundation in the kingdom. The commissioners were to investigate 'all Crimes, Defects, Abuses, Corruptions, Irregularitys and Enormitys' in the hospitals, and given full powers to deal with them, including if necessary the removal of 'any Master, Head, Governor, Officer or Officers'.[99] Although the Commission covered all royal hospitals, its only visible target was St Thomas's.

Thus by a strange irony, having struggled so hard to regain control of the hospital, Sir John Lawrence was now faced with an almost exact repetition of the events of

October/November 1683. In September the aldermen appointed a committee composed solely of St Thomas's governors 'to consider how farre the said Commission may affect the Rights and Interests of this City'.[100] The governors of St Thomas's prepared to defend their position, arguing that the Commission was invalid, because Edward VI's letters patent had left ultimate power over hospital affairs with the Court of Governors.[101] Yet there was an undeniable air of panic at St Thomas's. Samuel Smith, one of the hospital's new surgeons, beseeched Alderman John Wildman, a leading City Whig and a St Thomas's governor, to come to the assistance of 'a usefull and Antient Body of men almost ruind by some pretended Friends, and undermining enemyes', and so 'bridle the like arbitrary and despoticke practice Creept into the hospitall'.[102] Events were soon to render Smith's hysteria needless.

The Lords Commissioners of the Great Seal at first delayed and finally refused to pass the Commission of Visitation under the Seal. In a report delivered to King William on 31 December 1691, they argued against the Commission on a variety of technical and legal grounds.[103] But their diffidence was based above all on considerations of political prudence; such a Commission they argued, was 'Unpresidented, Arbitrary, of Dangerous consequence', and indeed

> may be of as evill consequence, as the late Commission in the late Reign [of James II] for the Visitation of Magdalen Coledg in Oxford, and in all probability would bee used by ill men to rayse Feares, Jealousyes, and discontents and cause a greater Fermentation amongst the Citizens of London and parts adjacent, than that did in the universityes.[104]

This was an amazing statement. It tells us much both of the government's fears of the City Whigs in the early 1690s, and the extent to which St Thomas's was seen as one of the focal points of London Whiggery.

The warnings of the Lords Commissioners were heeded. The King referred the 'legall part' of the report to the consideration of the Crown's law officers, but no further action was taken.[105] Early in the new year John Browne appealed directly to the Marquess of Carmarthen, the Tory

Lord President of the Council, to intervene on behalf of the surgeons. In a vituperative letter, he viciously denounced the governors and staff of St Thomas's as dissenters and republicans, that same breed of men who had 'made the best of Princes [Charles I], the celebrated Martyre of their inextricable malice'.[106] Browne's most splenetic outburst was reserved for the Lords Commissioners of the Great Seal, for they had advised the King 'to stand still with his arms claspt about him, whilst his enemyes are buffetting him'.[107]

But Browne was fighting a lost cause. Although there appears to have been a minor flurry of activity in August 1692, no action on his behalf was forthcoming from the King and his ministers.[108] In that same month, upon the death of Samuel Smith, Browne applied unsuccessfully to the St Thomas's governors for the vacancy; in 1699 he was still engaged in a solitary and forlorn battle for restoration.[109]

Sir John Lawrence survived just long enough to see off the renewed threat of royal intervention in St Thomas's affairs, for he died on 26 January 1692. It is in the figure of Sir John that the vicissitudes of St Thomas's hospital between 1683 and 1692 are best encapsulated. In the early 1680s he had used the hospital's patronage to foster dissent and Whiggery in Southwark. As a result he had been ejected in 1683, together with the many of the governors and staff. From 1689 to 1691 he led the struggle to reverse the actions of Charles II's commissioners, but by his zealous and pigheaded partisanship had helped to provoke the prospect of further Crown intervention. Above all he was responsible, more than any other, for ensuring that St Thomas's Hospital remained a Whig stronghold. When the governors met to elect Lawrence's successor in February 1692, it was fitting that they should choose Sir Robert Clayton, the most magnificent figure in London Whiggery.[110]

Conclusion

The events of 1683 to 1692 had shown that the London royal hospitals could not stand aloof from wider political developments. In October 1683, when the Corporation of London was dissolved, Charles II had also felt it necessary to intervene in the administration of the hospitals. The property they owned and the revenues they controlled gave the hospitals important local influence, an influence that the King would not allow to be exploited by his enemies. A Royal Commission was established to supervise the administration of the hospitals, ensure the loyalty of their governors and further the economic war against the dissenters. At St Thomas's Hospital, where the dominant group of Whig and Nonconformist governors had long worried the government, a severe purge of governors and staff ensued. Christ's Hospital was also badly hit by the Commissioners, but Bridewell was relatively unscathed. At St Bartholomew's Hospital, whose governors were fervently loyal to the Crown, there was no need for any action. However, it was Tory St Bartholomew's which was worst affected by royal intervention in the reign of James II, although that King's purge of Tory hospital presidents in 1687 was of less consequence than the purge of 1683. The Glorious Revolution led to a reversal of King James's intervention of 1687, and at St Thomas's it also eventually resulted in the overturning of all the Commission's actions since 1683. After a hard struggle St Thomas's and its patronage were regained by the Whigs in 1691, only for William III's government, fearful of Whig radicalism, to threaten further intervention in the hospital's affairs. That threat was seen off, and St Thomas's was to remain a bastion of London Whiggery. In contrast London's other great medical hospital, St Bartholomew's, was committed even more firmly to the Tories. In 1692 the contrast between the two hospitals was no better symbolized than in the figures of their respective presidents: at St Thomas's, Sir Robert Clayton, the Whig who had led the defence of the City's charter in 1683; at St Bartholomew's, Sir William Pritchard, who as Lord Mayor in 1682–3 had been Charles II's principal ally in gaining its surrender.

Notes

1. I would like to thank Mark Goldie, John Morrill, and Roy Porter for criticizing earlier drafts of this essay. I am also grateful to those who commented upon versions of this essay, which were read to seminars in Cambridge, Exeter, and London in 1986 and 1987.

2. For example, see Sir Norman Moore, *History of St Bartholomew's Hospital*, 2 vols (C. Arthur Pearson, London, 1918); F.G. Parsons, *History of St Thomas's Hospital*, 3 vols (Methuen, London, 1933–6); E.H. Pearce, *Annals of Christ's Hospital* (Hugh Rees, London 1901); E.G. O'Donoghue, *Bridewell Hospital*, 2 vols (Bodley Head, London, 1923–9), and *The Story of Bethlem Hospital* (T. Fisher, Unwin, London, 1914).

3. Paul Slack, 'Social policy and constraints of government, 1547–58', in Jennifer Loach and Robert Titler (eds), *The Mid-Tudor Polity c. 1540–1560* (Macmillan, London, 1980), 108–13.

4. Moore, *St Bartholomew's Hospital*, vol. 2, 182–7.

5. British Library Sloane MS 2728A, fos 2–3.

6. *Calendar of State Papers Domestic*, March-December 1678, 87–8; Pepys Library MS 2,612, fo. 721. The two medical hospitals had about 250 patients each at any one time.

7. St. Bartholomew's Hospital HB 1/9, fo. 141, Pepys Library MS 2,612, fo. 723. For St Thomas's, see p. 129.

8. Greater London Records Office H1/ST/A 91/5.

9. For the general political background, see J.R. Jones, *The First Whigs* (Oxford University Press, 1961).

10. G.R. Cragg, *Puritanism in the Period of the Great Persecution 1660–88* (Cambridge University Press, 1957), 24–6; John Miller, *Popery and Politics in England 1660–88* (Cambridge University Press, 1973), 189–95.

11. D.F. Allen, 'The Crown and the Corporation of London in the exclusion crisis', unpublished PhD thesis, University of Cambridge, 1978; A.G. Smith, 'London and the Crown, 1681–5', unpublished PhD thesis, University of Wisconsin, 1967.

12. Smith, 'London and the Crown', 285–309, 336–9.

13. Corporation of London Records Office Repertory 87, fos 86, 93.

14. Greater London Records Office H1/ST/A1/6, fo. 23.

15. Parsons, *St Thomas's Hospital*, vol. 2, 102; W.G. Bell, *The Great Plague of London in 1665* (Bodley Head, London, 1924), 70, 227–8. For general biographical details, see J.R. Woodhead, *The Rulers of London 1660–89* (London and Middlesex Archaeological Society, London, 1967), 106.

16. British Library Stowe MS 186, fos 5–9.

17. Tim Harris, *London Crowds in the Reign of Charles II* (Cambridge University Press, 1987), 178.

18. Bodleian MS Tanner 140, fo. 111.

19. British Library Sloane MS 2,728A, fo. 64, is a list of the hospital governors prior to the purge of 1683. Like most of the governors' lists, it was probably drawn up during the struggle for control of the hospital after 1689. Because of this, it only listed those governors still alive in 1689–90, and contains seventy-four names. However, the names of a further twenty-eight governors of 1683, who had died by 1690, have been discovered thanks to another list

in fos 55–6 of the same MS. This list dates from 1679, with additions for 1680 and 1681. From this second list, it has been deduced that the hospital had 130 governors in 1681.

20. The principal source for identifying political allegiance is the biographical data contained in Woodhead, *Rulers of London*. The *Dictionary of National Biography* and B.D. Henning (ed.), *The House of Commons 1660–90*, 3 vols (Secker & Warburg, London, 1983) were also consulted. Where these sources failed to identify the political allegiance of a governor, I have assumed that if he attended any hospital business after the purge of October 1683, then he was probably a Tory. Conversely, if a governor attended no hospital business during the rule of the commissioners but did so after 1688, I have assumed that he was a Whig ejected in 1683. This method is certainly not foolproof, and so the total figures should be treated with some caution. It should also be noted that the nature of the sources makes it easier to identify Tories than Whigs. There will be a full discussion of biographical methods and pitfalls in the relevant chapter of my PhD thesis.

21. Bodleian MS Tanner 140, fo. 111.

22. Anthony Wood, *Athenae Oxonienses*, éd. Philip Bliss, 4 vols (London, 1813–20), vol. 4, cols 541–4.

23. William Hughes, *Magistracy and Ministry, or a Rule for the Rulers and People's due Correspondence* (1652), 13, 20.

24. Wood, *Athenae*, vol. 4, col. 542.

25. See Hughes' pamphlet, *An Endeavour for Peace Among Protestants* (1680), which urged the comprehension of dissenters within the Church of England.

26. John Turner, *A Second Representation of the Hospitaller of St Thomas Southwark's Case* (1689), 5.

27. *Calendar of State Papers Domestic* July–September 1683, 235.

28. John Turner, *An Argument in Defence of the Hospitaller of St Thomas Southwark* (1689), 19.

29. Greater London Records Office H1/ST/E29/5, fos 228–30.

30. Henning, *The House of Commons*, vol. 1, 414.

31. Bodleian MS Tanner 140, fo. 111.

32. Greater London Records Office H1/ST/E29/5 fos 231–4.

33. *Calendar of State Papers Domestic*, October 1683–April 1684, 36.

34. Op. cit. January–June 1683, 10–11.

35. Op. cit. July–September 1683, 235.

36. Op. cit. October 1683–April 1684, 36.

37. Op. cit. 44–5.

38. Op. cit. 56. The commissioners are listed in St Bartholomew's Hospital Ha 1/7, fo. 137.

39. St. Bartholomew's Hospital Ha 1/7, fos 135–7 records the proceedings of the commissioners.

40. Smith, 'London and the Crown', 266; Harris, *London Crowds*, 210.

41. Other than Lawrence and the treasurer, we only know the

identity of eight of the ejected governors, who in 1688 wrote a memorial on behalf of the displaced officers. See British Library Sloane MS 2,728A, fo. 15.

42. Lists of the Commission governors can be found in British Library Sloane MSS 2,728A, fos 74–5, and 2,728B, fo. 214. The lists each contain approximately 140 names, with all but ten or so appearing in both lists. It is unlikely that so many governors were appointed at one time, so it probably includes all the governors appointed during the rule of the commissioners.

43. British Library Sloane MS 2,728A, fo.15.

44. Greater London Records Office H1/ST/A1/6, fos 27–9.

45. Bodleian MS Tanner 140, fos 112–13. The dismissal of the 'Brewers, Bakers, Artificers and others that sold provisions to the house for the use of the poore' is mentioned in British Library Sloane MS 2,728A, fo. 15.

46. See p. 135.

47. Turner, *Second Representation*, p. 7; Turner, *A Memorial Humbly Presented to the Right Honourable The Lord Chief Justice Of the King's-Bench In Behalf of the Hospitaller and His Friends* (1690), epistle dedicatory.

48. Woodhead, *Rulers of London*, 73; *Calendar of State Papers Domestic*, October 1683–April 1684, 36.

49. Guildhall Library MS 12,806/7, fos 495–9.

50. O'Donoghue, *Bridewell*, vol. 2, 159.

51. Nellie J.M. Kerling, 'The parish of St Bartholomew the Less', in Victor Cornelius Medvei and John L. Thornton (eds), *The Royal Hospital of St Bartholomew 1123–1973* (St Bartholomew's Hospital, London, 1974), 40–1. British Library Sloane MS 203, fo. 130, is a list of hospital governors in about 1682. It contains the names of 221 governors, of whom seventy-eight can be identified as Tories from the biographical sources cited in note 20. A further sixty-six governors can be labelled probable Tories on the basis of continued involvement in hospital business after 1683. Only ten of the governors can be identified as Whigs.

52. St Bartholomew's Hospital Ha 1/7, fo. 126.

53. Op. cit., fo. 169.

54. Op. cit., fo. 198.

55. Op. cit., fo. 302.

56. Op. cit., fos 172, 192.

57. Op. cit., fo. 162.

58. Op. cit., fos 195–9.

59. Op. cit., fo. 307.

60. J.R. Jones, *The Revolution of 1688 in England* (Weidenfeld & Nicolson, London 1972), 164.

61. St Bartholomew's Hospital Ha 1/7, fo. 208.

62. Guildhall Library MS 12,806/7, fos 780, 837.

63. Two of the governors definitely ejected in 1683 appear after March 1688 on the register of hospital takers-in, those governors

who supervised the admission of patients. Three other governors appear on this register after March 1688, having had nothing to do with the hospital since 1683. One of these was a Presbyterian. Greater London Records Office H1/ST/A62, fo. 46.

64. Jones, *Revolution of 1688*, 263.

65. Corporation of London Records Office Repertory 94, fos 38–9; St Bartholomew's Hospital MS Ha 1/7, fo. 320; Guildhall Library MS 12,806/7, fo. 879; O'Donoghue, *Bridewell*, vol. 2, 161.

66. Corporation of London Records Office MS 58.4.

67. British Library Sloane MS 2,728A, fo. 59.

68. Corporation of London Records Office MS 58.4.

69. Corporation of London Records Office Repertory 94, fo. 91.

70. For Turner's case, see the pamphlets cited in notes 26, 28, and 47.

71. Greater London Records Office H1/ST/A1/6, fo. 36; Public Records Office PC2/74, fos 82-3.

72. Greater London Records Office H1/ST/A1/6/2, fos 76 *passim*, for the committee's proceedings in 1689–90; British Library Sloane MS 2,728A, fo. 66, for its composition.

73. Greater London Records Office H1/ST/A1/6, fo. 33; Corporation of London Records Office Repertory 95, fo. 159.

74. For the main biographical sources, see note 20.

75. See Smith 'London and the Crown', Appendix, table 7, for a list of London Whigs against whom action was taken during Monmouth's rising.

76. G.S. De Krey, 'Political radicalism in London after the Glorious Revolution', *Journal of Modern History*, 55 (1983), 585–617, at p. 594. Another two of the Whig leaders were already governors of St Thomas's.

77. G.S. De Krey, *A Fractured Society* (Oxford University Press, 1985), 16.

78. British Library Sloane MS 2,728A, fo. 59.

79. Corporation of London Records Office Repertory 95, fo. 181; British Library Sloane MS 2,728B, fo. 178.

80. Corporation of London Records Office Repertory 95, fos 208, 305, 318, 324; St Bartholomew's Hospital Ha 1/8, fos 47, 58, 60.

81. British Library Sloane MS 2,728A, fo. 61. For Lawrence's reply, see British Library Sloane MS 2,728B, fo. 120.

82. Corporation of London Records Office Repertory 95, fos 233-5; British Library Sloane MS 2,728A, fos 2-3.

83. Greater London Records Office H1/ST/A1/6, fos 33-4.

84. Op. cit. fo. 36; British Library Sloane MS 2,728A, fo. 63.

85. These three were Michael Court and Thomas Elton, senior surgeons, and William Pepper, junior surgeon.

86. Greater London Records Office H1/ST/A1/6, fo. 25.

87. Op. cit., fo. 34.

88. Greater London Records Office H1/ST/A6/2, fo. 87.

89. In 1699 two of the surgeons resorted to fisticuffs while

attending patients, because of a dispute over seniority. The senior surgeon marched in front of the others at the Easter Spittle Sermon, given for the aldermen and the hospital governors. See E.M. McInnes, *St Thomas' Hospital* (George Allen & Unwin, London, 1963), 65.

90. Greater London Records Office H1/ST/A1/6, fo. 35.

91. Op. cit., fo. 37.

92. *Dictionary of National Biography*.

93. Greater London Records Office H1/ST/A91/9.

94. Public Records Office PC2/74, fos 210–11.

95. Op. cit., fo. 213.

96. British Library Harleian MS 6,190 is a register of the seamen treated in the hospital between 1689 and 1693. These numbered 1,943.

97. For William III and the City Whigs, see De Krey, *Fractured Society*, 61–3, and 'Political radicalism', 599–600. E.L. Ellis, 'William III and the politicians', in Geoffrey Holmes (ed.), *Britain after the Glorious Revolution* (Macmillan, London, 1969), 115–34, gives a succinct account of the King's relationship with the parties.

98. For the Act for reversing the *quo warranto*, see De Krey, *Fractured Society*, 64. The Act restored all charter officers deposed at the time of the *quo warranto*, but confirmed in their places those appointed thereafter.

99. Corporation of London Records Office Misc. MS 27.14.

100. Corporation of London Records Office Repertory 95, fo. 341.

101. Greater London Records Office H1/ST/A91/7; Pepys Library MS 2612, fos 730c–e.

102. British Library Sloane MS 1,731A, fo. 56.

103. Pepys Library MS 2,612, fos 730e–i. The report also appears, together with John Browne's comments, in British Library Egerton MS 3383, fos 108–15.

104. Op. cit., fos 111-12. For the Magdalen College affair of 1687, see Jones, *Revolution of 1688*, 119–21.

105. British Library Sloane MS 2,728A, fo. 8.

106. British Library Egerton MS 3,383, fo. 108.

107. Op. cit., fo. 112.

108. Greater London Records Office H1/ST/A1/6, fo. 42.

109. Op. cit., fo. 68.

110. Op. cit., fo. 40.

6

The gift relation: philanthropy and provincial hospitals in eighteenth-century England

Roy Porter

Laurence Sterne's *A Sentimental Journey* (1760) opens with a sentimental yet disturbing vignette about giving. Solicited in Calais for alms by a mendicant monk, the hero resolves in his head not to give, on the grounds that stout Protestant Englishmen properly offer charity only to those who 'eat the bread of their own labour' not those who 'eat the bread of other people's'. Yet he longs to give – 'my heart smote me'.[1] His emotions gain the day, but with a whimsically arbitrary outcome; the hero gives the monk his snuff-box, and they part soul mates in sentimental floods of tears.

The cameo captures the equivocations of charity in Georgian England. Philanthropy was assuredly in fashion. As Henry Fielding put it in 1749, 'Charity is the very characteristic virtue at this time' – adding rather uncharitably, 'I believe we may challenge the whole world to parallel the examples we have of late given of this noble, this Christian virtue'.[2] Yet the age was also perturbed by its enigmas. If charity sprang from spontaneous feeling, what if the heart – as with the heart of Sterne's hero – was wayward in its objects? If the heart seemed to have reasons of which the reason knew nothing? Both sentimentalists and dismal economists could foresee the generous impulse opening a Pandora's box of evils. And so the Georgians preoccupied themselves with plotting the proper pathways from impulse to action, from causes to consequences, weighing good intentions alongside value for money. Springing from the heart, benevolence could all too easily be wasteful or even counterproductive, demoralizing to the recipients, and the dupe of fraud. Yet however precarious and liable to abuse, charity was something that had to be dispensed, rather than dispensed with. It was after all the cardinal Christian virtue, the hallmark of humanity and, not least, of the gentleman, a generosity soaring above the sordid miserliness of the vulgar, above the institutionalized, anonymous, halfpenny dribblings of the parish poor law.[3]

Thus aware of Sterne's dilemma, the Georgians hoped to sail the course between the Scylla of sentiment and the Charybdis of calculation, fusing the heart of generosity with the brain of utility into practical outlets. One of the most popular instruments devised for this purpose – pretty much a Georgian invention – was the voluntary hospital; or, as John Aikin rather insistently called it in his *Thoughts on hospitals* (1771), the 'infirmary', thus underlining its specifically medical nature and clearly distancing it from the traditional association of 'hospital' with 'almshouse', with its connotations of poor law provision for indigent paupers.[4] In this paper I shall explore the resonances of giving, and of receiving, as they formed the order of the Georgian provincial infirmary, viewed both ethnographically, as a symbolic meaning system, and practically, as a microeconomy of exchange; and I shall do so in the light of Ferdnand Braudel's dictum 'he who gives, dominates'. This is not a study of the workings of the eighteenth-century hospital; rather an analysis of its underlying ideology.

If my rehearsal of contemporary rhetoric and rationalizations for charity to the sick sound hackneyed, echoing soporific platitudes, this is (I fear) as it ought to be, and forms an integral part of the story. For there was indeed a striking uniformity to the provincial infirmary. The early foundations in the 1730s – Winchester, Bristol, Exeter, York, etc. – were cloned again and again throughout the nation; Bath, Northampton, Worcester, Shrewsbury, and Liverpool had followed before 1750, and then in the second half of the century, Newcastle, Manchester, Gloucester, Cambridge, Salisbury, Leeds, and many others followed suit.[5] Whereas there were none in 1735, sixteen provincial voluntary hospitals existed by 1760 and thirty-eight by 1800, and all followed the same model, framed similar rules, and made identical appeals to the passions, piety, prudence, and pockets of the locals. Indeed, the first founder, the Reverend Alured Clarke, was to repeat himself when he was ecclesiastically translated from

Winchester to Exeter; and partly because his benevolent schemes were fanfared throughout the pages of the *Gentleman's Magazine*, Clarke's own rules and persuasives were taken up verbatim as blueprints across the nation.[6] For example, when the Salop Infirmary was established in 1747, the governors recommended[7]:

> For the better conducting it, the Rules and Orders drawn up for the government of *Winchester Hospital*, which are published by Dr. Alured Clarke, may be consulted; and what further information can be had from the Hospitals and Infirmaries in London, will be ready to be laid before the Subscribers for their consideration; from which helps it will be easy to draw out such a plan, as (with the blessing of God) will not fail to answer the charitable ends intended.

In points of detail the provincial infirmaries evolved differentially during the century, some sprouting fever wings, some lunatic asylums, bath-houses, electric machines, and others chapels, but the vital force remained the reciprocity of giving and receiving. For the annual infirmary sermons (perhaps delivered to Hogarthian sleeping congregations), dinners, and public collections at the assizes and the races, all helped keep the guineas jingling in. Only exceptionally did the Georgian infirmary suffer financial collapse or a major crisis of public confidence.

If infirmary publicity promoted in sermons, annual reports, and the newspapers, wears a familiar and bland face, that is precisely because it was meant to be uplifting, uncontroversial, and soothing. The hospital was there to heal the sick; but it was intended to function as a social balm as well. Throughout the Tudor and Stuart age, the springs of doing good had become polluted through sectarian theological warfare (after all, the Reformation had put the very doctrine of good works under a cloud, as a Popish deviation, and had asset-stripped much of the medieval machinery of organized charity).[8] Hence charitable action in the seventeenth century frequently had a sectarian sting in the tail. When early Stuart corporations funded town preachers, it would be seen by Laudians as a Puritan gesture against the hierarchy. The Georgians by contrast breathed a sigh of relief to discover in the infirmary a vehicle for practical benevolence which seemed proof against theological sniping (more so, for example, than smallpox inoculation), and which did not arouse the same sociopolitical anxieties as schemes to teach the poor to write, or workhouses, or model colonies abroad. It seemed Alexander Pope's pieties came true[9]:

> In Faith and Hope the world will disagree,
> But all mankind's concern is Charity.

Georgian opinion vested great faith in the hospital as a symbolic clasping of hands between the social ranks. Capitalism was arguably constantly widening the gulf between masters and men, and all the more so as the science of political economy replaced the ethics of the 'moral economy'. Recognizing the perils of naked class antagonisms, the propertied, as E.P. Thompson has argued, fabricated elaborate and spectacular rituals of paternalistic care – specious, but theatrically effective.[10] Thus the severe – indeed increasingly severe – justice and majesty of the law were tempered by displays of the quality of mercy; wage labour was to be softened once in a while by the harvest supper and yuletide largesse. An act of conspicuous, self-congratulatory, stage-managed *noblesse oblige* similarly underlay the infirmary. Poverty, malnutrition, premature ageing, occupational accidents, and diseases would remain the abiding realities of life for the labouring classes, as would the coercive, police functions of the poor law for ensuring a tractable labour force. But the infirmary threw a cloak of charity over the bones of poverty and naked repression.[11] It enabled the polite and propertied to pose as tender souls, as those, indeed, who were fired by a generous disdain for the flinty provisions of the poor law, the workhouse, and the bridewell. Alured Clarke at Winchester, and all those who subsequently parrotted and paraphrased him, dismissed care for the sick in the workhouse as inadequate to meet the need. Subscribers clearly sought a conspicuous monument of prestigious charity, distinct from the tainting and compulsory housekeeping of the poor law system. By patronizing voluntary hospitals as a separate additional stratum on top of the parish system, donors got the best of both worlds. In the poor law workhouse they showed the hand that disciplined; in the infirmary, the hand that gave, for in the infirmary, as Bishop Isaac Maddox, founder of the Worcester Infirmary, put it in 1743, 'the poor and the rich meet together'.[12]

The infirmary was thus in some measure to close the rift, or at least to paper over the cracks, between patricians and plebeians. But no less important a function was that of healing the wounds within the propertied classes themselves, as Maddox acknowledged in the same sermon when he referred to the 'asperities' so dangerous in civil society which would be smoothed down by 'mutual intercourse in works of charity', providing a 'friendly cement'.[13] Contemporaries were perturbed by the tensions in what Holmes and Speck have dubbed 'the divided society'.[14] In the Stuart century the governing classes had been split by struggles between Anglican, Papist, and Puritan, between Royalist and Roundhead; by the early eighteenth century these had become the dogfights of Hanoverian *versus* Jacobite, Whig *versus* Tory, established church *versus* dissenter, ministerialist *versus* the backwoods squirearchy, town *versus* country, landed *versus* moneyed wealth and trade. Opinion leaders – pre-eminently Addison and Steele in the *Spectator* – were making a concerted appeal for the ruling orders to close ranks and pull together (Mr Spectator's own club being the epitome of this, where all gentlemen of good will – Tory and Whig, ancients and moderns, landed and trading – could smoke a pipe of peace together). The hospital was promoted as precisely the engine to unify and integrate the propertied of every hue and all the gradations of rank. Thus in 1766, making an appeal for an infirmary in Leicester, William Watts claimed it would help quieten 'the vile, and most Unchristian Spirit of Party itself'.[15] But the religious hatchet also should be buried. The governors' publicity for the Devon and Exeter Infirmary thus argued that it would 'unite Good Men of all Denominations more firmly with us in a common cause',[16] and Joseph Priestley made the same point quite explicitly in his 1768 sermon on behalf of the Leeds Infirmary[17]:

It is a recommendation of this scheme, that the benefits of it are not confined to any particular sect or party in religion; but that it is equally open to all who may stand in need of it. It has therefore a natural claim to the patronage and support of all those who make pretensions to catholicism; and who while they profess to be *Christians* forget not that they are *men*, but bear an affectionate regard to all their brethren of mankind, however distinguished by religious epithets and denominations.

The hope that men of good will would bury their differences and remember the good Samaritan was in fact often realized. Thus at Northampton the two leading promoters of the hospital, working cheek by jowl, were the Anglican, Dr James Stonhouse, and the eminent dissenter, Philip Doddridge[18]; while at Exeter and elsewhere, both the Anglican and the dissenting clergy agreed to hold collections at their services (infirmary doors were of course to be open to all denominations).[19] And in Bristol, newspapers were pleased to report that subscribers to the infirmary included 'Persons of all Persuasions'.[20]

Of course, so entrenched and spiteful were local factions that such reconciliations through giving were not achieved everywhere. In Leicester, for example, the hospital pressure group came to be identified with Whiggish country gentlemen, who used it as a vehicle for their opposition to the oligarchic Tory corporation.[21] In fact, the Leicester corporation gave not a penny towards the founding of the infirmary, which was managed by a cabal of prominent Whigs – the Duke of Montagu, the Earl of Stamford, and Lord Wentworth. Something rather similar transpired at Exeter. There the City Hospital had been founded in 1701, as a poor law almshouse under the auspices of the corporation. A rival infirmary (i.e. medical hospital), the Devon and Exeter, was then launched in 1741, following the promptings of country gentlemen and leading clergy, especially Alured Clarke. Fierce contention flared for a few years, as is described by a contemporary surgeon, Bartholomew Parr[22]:

The contest between the two institutions was carried on for some time with unabating rancour. The Chamber [i.e. the City Council] subscribing £100 to one annually. The country gentlemen and the Church as liberally supported the other. The surgeons supplied in the County Hospital their own dressings and the apothecaries of the town their own medicines. The Chamber published a plan of Exeter which showed their favourite institution with a prospect of fields and a dairy maid milking a cow, while that of the County Hospital displayed the graveyard and a funeral procession.

The City Hospital eventually collapsed, and the Devon and Exeter went on to thrive.

Factions also occasionally arose within the infirmaries. Thus a movement gained ground in the 1760s at the Bristol Infirmary for remunerating a clergyman for his services.[23] In 1773 a decision was taken to salary an Anglican chaplain out of general infirmary funds, which provoked a threatened walkout by Quaker and dissenter subscribers before a compromise was reached. And at the Manchester Infirmary a secession actually occurred. As Pickstone and Butler have shown, by the late 1780s a radical and Whiggish ginger group amongst the subscribers was trying to make its presence felt, by moving that the infirmary should reach out more into the community, in particular by establishing a lying-in service. In retaliation, the leading lights of the honorary medical staff, all Tories – Charles White and his son, and Edward Hall and his son – quit the institution and set up their own rival, the St Mary's Lying-in Hospital.[24]

These instances are however exceptional. But they attest to the corrosiveness of local passions, and, in doing so, indicate the wisdom of infirmary promoters in making their institutions as accommodating and ecumenical as possible, and point to the broad success of the infirmary movement in reconciling the divided society by gift-relations.[25] For infirmaries actually became foci of civic loyalties, escaping the opprobrium of cabal warfare and the worst accusations of jobbery and nepotism which dogged the Georgian corporation and many long-standing charitable trusts.[26] Whereas in London the multiplicity of hospitals led each to acquire some colour of party loyalty – thus St Thomas's was visibly pro-Whig and dissenter, whereas Bart's was high church and Tory, as Craig Rose's preceding chapter shows – the fact that provincial towns housed only a single infirmary encouraged locals to sink their differences. Thereby the infirmary became a proud manifestation of civic spirit and achievement in an age when, with the urban economy booming, citizens could afford to give more to charity, while signalling that they were not boorishly money-mad but participants in a cosmopolitan emulative and fashionable culture of science, benevolence, and humanity, of which the infirmary was a prize bloom.[27]

The infirmary was also an expression of a wider movement for institutional renewal. Traditional institutions – Parliament, the established church, the corporations, urban, and medical – had grown hidebound, torpid, oligarchic, unable to meet the challenges of the emerging new society (for example, in expanding towns the demand for better paving, lighting, and drainage). Free associations of influential public-spirited gentlemen and citizens were coalescing to meet these needs. The voluntary hospital was just such a creation, owing little to official initiatives, local or central. Thus, for example, of the £4,000 or so subscribed to the Newcastle Infirmary, just £100 came from the corporation.[28] The infirmary thereby marks pregnant new allegiances of the polite and moneyed, brought together in the name of giving.

What form, then, did the infirmary actually take? Its key features were that it mobilized collective, not individual, charity, and giving by the living rather than through bequest. The main pattern of charity established in the middle ages, and continued thereafter, was the endowment set up by individual munificence, often perpetuating the family name, usually not taking effect till after the donor's death, and frequently with a view to settling accounts with God.[29] Most Tudor and Stuart schools and almshouses were of that kind. But hardly any Georgian infirmaries were. Guy's is the outstanding exception. But the only provincial hospital following that pattern is Addenbrooke's in Cambridge, and the fact that it was set up by private bequest surely explains its uniquely sickly early career – established in 1719, it did not open its doors till 1766.[30]

Rather, the Georgian infirmary, like most other Georgian charities, operated on a kind of joint stock principle. The donors were numerous; they were typically the living (though of course bequests were gratefully accepted as well); and they were encouraged to be long-term subscribers, giving, say, two guineas a year for life. This arrangement amounted to a clever and extremely successful instrument of charity. Ever suspicious of human nature, the Georgians recognized that the lump-sum bequest from an individual almost inevitably fell prey, after his death, to misappropriation, malversation, or embezzlement – in short, as Joseph Priestley put it,[31] 'to those abuses which we see, by lamentable experience, never fail to creep into the disposal of fixed revenues'. But the infirmary's magic formula was proof against that. Because it was by the living, giving purchased a stake in the infirmary's management and resources. A substantial donation (at the Salop Infirmary the minimum was 20 guineas) made one a manager or trustee, with a right to sit on the board of governors; a smaller offering – a couple of guineas a year was typical – bought lesser rights to nominate in- or outpatients. Thus the simple device of attaching rights, privileges, and duties to philanthropy ensured that the donor's interest lay in avoiding mismanagement of his own moneys. That this was intended as a prophylactic against corruption was clearly spelt out at the time, as by the managers at the Salop Infirmary[32]:

> To prevent any misapplication of the Charity, the government of it must be placed in the hands of the *Principal Benefactors* to it, who will of consequence be most interested in its success; and a state of the accounts must be published from time to time, for the satisfaction of all the *Contributors*.

And because the institution depended on repeated annual gifts, regular and careful housekeeping was essential. Thus the cunning of the infirmary gift-relation lay in the fact that charitable giving was not the discharging of a responsibility once and for all, but the acquisition of one. The donation of money merely opened the doors to the donation of time, expertise, and involvement.

Who then was it who gave? It was essential to the wider social purposes of the infirmary that a broad social spectrum should be encouraged to give; the more donors, the more the community consensus, and the healthier the revenues. Community pockets were tapped in an inventive variety of ways, anticipating later 'flag days'. Annual charity sermons were preached, followed by silver collections, which often raised up to £100; routine Sunday church collections were sometimes earmarked for the infirmary. Collections were held at the assizes, assemblies, and the races. Special gala concerts and charitable theatre performances were mounted – thus from the beginning the Birmingham Music Festival was a fundraiser for the General Hospital.[33] The secretary of the Worcester Infirmary personally rode round the county on special fund-raising tours. And, to reach the lower ranks, collecting boxes were padlocked to the walls of inns, and house-to-house collections were even staged.[34] Apparently gifts did indeed flow in from people not specially affluent, and hospitals commonly welcomed benefactions in kind rather than in cash. The benefaction book at Northampton includes, for example, the gift of a large knife and fork from a Mr Bignall, and a candle box and a dripping pan from another donor, both quite possibly small tradesmen or shopkeepers.[35]

But who gave the princely sums? A well-established view amongst historians of hospitals attributes the greatest generosity to the middle classes, proverbially rising. As Leader and Snell put it in their account of the Sheffield Infirmary,[36]

> The Hospitals and Infirmaries founded during the 18th century owed their birth, not so much to the great landowners as to the prosperous manufacturers and merchants. It was a popular movement not an aristocratic one.

In a more general context this view has been supported by David Owen[37]:

> Associated philanthropy was, in a large measure, middle class in its support and Puritan in its temper . . . donors came overwhelmingly from trade and commerce rather than from the great families.

But these conclusions seem dubious for the infirmaries, particularly at the time of the great fund-raising drives needed to get them off the ground. Certainly their publicity targeted overwhelmingly on the landed orders and the upper clergy, as witness this appeal for the Norfolk and Norwich in 1744[38]:

> Let me therefore propose to your consideration, amongst other Motives to this Charitable Undertaking, the following: – THAT Norfolk is abundantly able to provide for

the Support of this Charity by Voluntary Contributions, and which therefore would be burdensome to NONE, but highly beneficial to MANY: – THAT we have several Noble Families and Gentlemen of large Estates and Influence, who would, as we may justly hope, be filled with a charming Emulation to deserve the Regards of their County by a distinguishing Benevolence on this occasion; whose skill is to direct, – whose Bounty to feed, – whose Example to dignifie and recommend this much-wanted Charity, all incourage us to hope for the happiest success.

The landed classes were indeed prominent in all the stages of seeding the infirmaries. Thus the foundation meeting of the Gloucester General Infirmary in 1754 was attended, so the newspapers reported, by 'the nobility, gentry and clergy of the county'.[39] The composition of the steering committee for the Norfolk and Norwich Hospital in 1770 consisted entirely of the landed and the higher clergy, i.e.

the Earl of Rosebery, the Earl of Albemarle, the Earl of Oxford, the Earl of Buckingham, Viscount Townshend, Lord Walpole, the Bishop of Norwich, Sir Edward Astley, Bart., Thomas de Grey, Esqre., Edward Bacon, Esqre., and William Fellowes, Esqre.[40]

Similarly, the list of governors of the Nottingham General Hospital for 1782 was headed by[41]:

The Most Noble Henry Fines Pelham Clinton, Duke of Newcastle, Lord Lieutenant of the County.
The Most Noble William Henry Cavendish Bentinck, Duke of Portland.
His Grace the Lord Archbishop of York.
The Right Honourable Henry, Lord Middleton.
Sir George Saville, Bart.,

and so forth. And Sir Francis Hill's verdict on the Lincoln County Hospital is that[42]

apart from the mayor and aldermen, who were governors *ex officio*, the hospital was wholly in the hands of the gentry and clergy. An annual sermon was preached in aid of it at the cathedral, at which ladies or gentlemen solicited contributions, and an annual charitable assembly was held for it in race week.

Not surprisingly, then, the big money came from the grandees. Take the Salisbury Infirmary, an institution which probably would not have been founded at all without a handsome aristocratic donation. When Lord Feaversham died in 1763, he bequeathed £500 'to the first infirmary that should be established in the County of Wilts, within five years of his decease'.[43] Acting on this spur, the city corporation immediately wrote to Lord Pembroke, Lord Radnor, and the Bishop of Salisbury, to get plans moving. Similarly, at the founding of the Nottingham General Hospital, the Hon. Henry Cavendish gave, anonymously, a staggering £6,337; the Duke of Newcastle gave £300, as did the Duke of Portland; whereas the largest local employer, the opulent millowner Richard Arkwright, gave £200.[44] Likewise when the Cornwall Infirmary was floated in 1799, the Prince of Wales gave £500, the Duke of Leeds and the Earl of Mount Edgecombe both £200, but none of the local tin and copper mining companies – surely the largest beneficiaries of the institution – gave more than 50 guineas.[45]

Why was this? It is partly because the grandees in general had more to give. It is importantly also because the infirmary movement, though building in town centres, was, both in inspiration and in actuality, very much a 'county' movement, galvanizing the local community at large and commonly involving the quite specific provision that the infirmary was not to be restricted to the sick poor resident in the home parish or town, but was to fling its doors wide open to the sick from everywhere – a 'generous' gesture of great benefit to the county. Thus the very masthead of the Sheffield General Infirmary stated that it was 'For the Reception of Sick and Lame Poor of any County'.[46] Indeed, a large proportion of the infirmaries either included the name of their county in their title – the Devon and Exeter Infirmary, the Norfolk and Norwich Hospital, the Salop Infirmary, the Durham County, the Lincoln County – or were known as 'general' hospitals (e.g. the Leeds General, the Sheffield General), the word 'general' signalling that the institution was not restricted, as were the poor law medical services, to labourers with a settlement in the home parish. In the voluntary infirmary the passport securing entry was not the parish settlement but the admission letter of the subscriber.

Moreover, the conspicuous show of *noblesse oblige* stemming from giving and serving was a highly effective means of asserting grandee cultural hegemony. David Cannadine has rightly stressed the eagerness of the Victorian aristocracy to serve as patrons of multitudes of good causes and local voluntary associations; as their economic and political grip on the nation slowly relaxed, cultural dominion came to count for more.[47] But in doing so, they were only sitting in seats already warmed by their grandfathers. The Duke of Portland was one of the founding fathers of the Nottingham General Hospital. In 1944 the Duke of Portland was still the president of what was still the voluntary hospital.

The landed classes were thus prominent patrons of the infirmaries. The Anglican clergy likewise sought to seal the bond between healing and holiness, by playing an active role. Several infirmaries owed their existence to clerical enthusiasm; both the Winchester and the Devon and Exeter arose largely through the energies of Alured Clarke, while Bishop Maddox founded the Worcester; and it is noteworthy how many cathedral cities got their infirmary in the first wave of foundations. Worcester, Hereford, Exeter, Salisbury, Winchester, all built their hospitals long before big, prosperous mercantile Hull, which had to wait until 1782, or Sheffield, which had no hospital till 1797. By contrast, the medical professions were perhaps less conspicuous in the launching of infirmaries than one might have supposed, confirming the impression that hospitals sprang more from a lay desire rooted in the community to generate appropriate charity than from strict evaluations of overwhelming medical need or even from the professional ambitions of the practitioners. Rather few infirmaries owed their origin to the campaigning zeal of practitioners (the Birmingham General, promoted by Dr Ash, is one exception).[48] But once an infirmary was launched, the medical staff took their place alongside the donors, wedded to charity not profit. It was the universal practice that the physicians and surgeons should be honorary, giving their services freely (though commonly they received a token honorarium). Infirmary rules often spelt this out: 'No fee or reward of the least kind shall be given to any person belonging to the hospital on any occasion' commanded one of the by-laws of the Devon and Exeter.[49] That the upper echelons of the medical staff should have been eager to serve *gratis* is no surprise. For, on the one hand, as Holmes and Loudon have argued, by the mid-eighteenth century, provincial practitioners were far more prosperous than ever; they could afford a generous philanthropic gesture.[50] While on the other, their 'gentlemanly' status in the community was still, however, somewhat less than assured, and they were in danger of being looked upon as a class of superior tradesmen; in such circumstances, an honorary appointment to a hospital would help elevate a practitioner into the genteel bracket as well as affording him close contact with his betters and the prospect of new lucrative high-class custom from the subscribers.

Having discussed who gave, I turn to the question of why they gave. The professed motives were many, varied, and overlapping. Everyone who argued the cause of charity stressed the pole star of duty – duty to God, duty to humanity. As the Revd Isaac Maddox put it in 1743, neatly dovetailing both: 'It is a *Christian* duty no less than a *social obligation of citizenship* to relieve the distress wrought by sickness and poverty.'[51] In the classical mode of Enlightenment utilitarian piety, it was also suggested that giving today was in fact a form of investment for the hereafter. Confirming this, one of the favourite texts used for hospital sermons was Psalm xli, 1, 'Blessed is the man that provideth for the sick and needy, the Lord shall deliver him in the time of trouble', a sentiment endorsed by Bishop Edmund Gibson, who preached in 1716 that 'whatever is laid out in Charity, God accounts an Offering and a Loan to himself: and accordingly he engaged to repay it'.[52] 'These poor people', Bishop Maddox assured his congregation, 'cannot recompense you; but you *will be recompensed at the resurrection of the just*'.[53]

But if charity was a duty, it was also a pleasure. The egotistical joys of giving were not denied or found embarrassing by the Georgians. Individually they liked to savour what the *Gentleman's Magazine* in 1732 called 'the most lasting, valuable and exquisite pleasure' of charity.[54] And collectively they plumed themselves that in giving so unstintingly they thereby proved themselves more civilized, sensitive, and tender, than their forebears or, doubtless, their inferiors. As the Annual Report of the Leeds Infirmary expressed it in 1784, the generosity of donors proved that 'the charity of Mankind . . . has been progressive, and reflects peculiar Lustre on the present Period'.[55] Joseph Priestley argued that in giving freely we 'reap all the advantages of the real refinements and true polish of the present age',[56] and, in a similar vein, William Watts urged his Leicester citizens, 'we are called to be charitable in an age, and nation, and instance, in which Charity abounds', in acts of benevolence in which 'public and private good are most intimately mixed'.[57]

Duty and pleasure, but also prudence. As the future Archbishop Secker – himself trained as a doctor – put that trinity: 'Religion, humanity, common Prudence, loudly require us to rescue' the sick poor.[58] The appeal to give from reasons of mercantilist self-interest was compelling. The sick poor could not afford medical treatment, or, as Bishop Maddox stressed, at best they went to quacks who were likely to disable them permanently. But they were the nation's workforce. If kept from work through disease or injury, the loss of their labour represented a direct debit to the community, with the risk of further charges if they and their families fell on to the parish. It was false economy not to help restore them to labour as speedily as possible. Thus, as Priestley phrased it, in the light of these arguments, the infirmary was 'the cheapest of all charities, the most great good being done with the least expense'.[59] The economics of the matter seemed decisive; infirmary treasurers calculated that the average cost of an inpatient amounted to about £3 12s. (these figures are from the Northampton Infirmary),[60] whereas at the beginning of the century the Quaker philanthropist John Bellers had calculated that the death of a labouring man, capable of bearing children, represented a capital loss to the community of some £200.[61]

Moreover, giving to the hospital meant saving in an additional way, for the hospital was represented as highly efficient on account of economies of scale. More of the sick poor could receive treatment there for less outlay, as compared with outdoor relief or one-off parish action. This persuasive argument runs like a watermark through the propaganda of the voluntary hospitals. Thus, noting that the poor, as much as we are apt to overlook them, are a very necessary and useful Part of the Community, nor ought it to be forgotten that to the Sweat of their Brows, and to the labour of their Hands, it is owing, that the Rich enjoy the Accommodation of Ease and Pleasure

the managers of the Nottingham General Hospital went on to argue how economically they could be relieved in hospitals[62]:

It has been laid down as Matter of Fact, confirmed by Experience, that distressed Objects are taken care of in Infirmaries, for a tenth Part of what must necessarily be spent for them at their own Habitations: so that the same Contributions which if disposed of separately, and in a private Manner would barely be sufficient for the Relief of Forty or Fifty Persons, when collected together and providently Managed, will answer the Distress of three or four hundred. And what is still more, supposing this Collection to be doubled, it will then extend to the Relief not of twice only, but of three Times the Number. For the larger the Contribution is upon the whole, the more is the Expense of each Patient abated.

Though all this had been said long before and more briefly by the patriarch of the movement, Alured Clarke: 'For a thousand persons will be relieved here at a less expense, than would be required for an hundred in the ordinary way of giving Alms.'[63]

Charity must come from the heart. But, the Georgian *Homo economicus* never tired of reminding himself, erratic, impulsive, blind benevolence would do more harm than good. Give thoughtlessly, warned Joseph Priestley, and[64]

with the best intention in the world, you may be doing nothing better than encouraging idleness, profligacy and imposture: but in the cases for which this infirmary is provided, there can be no imposition, and avarice has none of its usual paltry excuses to avail itself of.

There is no denying, as Lewis and Williams stressed,[65] that personal, *ad hominem* charity flourished in Hanoverian times. Yet as Sterne's *Sentimental Journey* suggests, there was also a rising horror against personal mendicancy, no sympathy for the old Popish image of the holy beggar, and a great terror of being duped by imposters (newspapers often carried warning stories of fraudulent beggars at large). These fears were crystallized by Bishop Maddox[66]:

> The more difficult it is to distinguish real from pretended objects of charity; and the greater inconveniencies arise from encouraging laziness and debauchery, under the appearance of distress, the more requisite it is to employ the strictest caution, that the clamorous and unworthy may not eat the bread of the poor; no idleness and imposture riot in that relief, which is justly due to actual want and sickness.

The great virtue of the hospital, by contrast, was that it institutionalized an effective, double-sifting procedure, to ensure that charity was properly dispensed, and thus was neither demoralizing nor wasteful, but rather expended on worthy objects for tangible benefits. For on the one hand there was a medical screening process, which barred patients suffering from chronic, terminal, or infectious conditions, for which the hospital could do nothing. As the Salop Infirmary rules put it[67]:

> that no woman big with child, no child under seven years of age (except in extraordinary cases such as Fractures, Stone or where Couching, Trepanning or Amputation are necessary), no persons disordered in their senses, suspected to have the small-pox or other infectious distempers, having habitual Ulcers, Cancers not admitting of Operation, epileptic and convulsive Fits, consumptive Coughs and Consumptions, or Dropsies in their last stages, in a dying condition, or judged incurable, be admitted as In-patients.

An embargo which sometimes had seemingly heartless consequences – 'Margaret Barnfield rejected as a patient being in a dying condition with dropsy and Gutta Serena'[68] – but which was designed to maximize bed-room for conditions which could profitably be treated – scurvy, abscesses, burns, skin complaints, leg ulcers, rheumatism, broken limbs, and the like.

And, on the other hand, there was the personal test. Patients were expected to be known to, and scrutinized by, the subscriber nominating them, to ensure that they indeed fell within the intended clientele, i.e. the labouring poor, being neither frauds, nor those who could afford to pay for their own treatment (for that would be taking bread out of the mouths of the physicians), nor the domestic servants of gentlemen who ought to foot the bill themselves (though rules against admitting the personal servants of subscribers tended to become relaxed in the course of time).

Ensuring strict propriety of admission was a constant headache. As the governors of the Norfolk and Norwich Hospital complained in 1788[69]:

> It is earnestly requested that every gentleman would inform himself of the circumstances of the person he recommends, as several have been admitted into the Hospital, of ability, it is believed, to have paid for their cure; whilst others have endeavoured to get admission whose circumstances have been known to be good; and some have made pecuniary offers to the Faculty for their attendance and skill, provided they would not oppose their admission in the Hospital. The injury the Charity must sustain if attempts of this sort are not speedily crushed, is too obvious to be insisted on, not to mention the injustice of breaking in upon the private practice and emoluments of many gentlemen in the profession of Physic and Surgery in the country.

Nevertheless the principle of individual charity, filtered through appropriate tests, absolutely matched the mood of the times. For the personal touch was vital, since, as Priestley told potential subscribers, the nominated patients 'will be your neighbours and acquaintances, in whose afflictions you will have previously sympathized and in whose relief you can heartily rejoice . . . you soon see the effect of your benevolence'.[70]

What, then, were the sick to do in return for being on the receiving end of the gift relation? How were they to perform 'gratitude'? First, patients were to be obedient and docile. Every hospital had its elaborate decalogue of house rules. At the Salop Infirmary two lists were posted on the walls, '*What*

The Patient May Expect' and *'What The Charity Requires'*, the latter far longer and including bans on cursing, gambling, smoking, going out without leave, or smuggling in hard liquor, and an absolute prohibition upon the mingling of male and female patients.[71] Patients could expect little say in their treatment. In his pioneering *Medical Ethics*, Thomas Percival explained that the sick poor in hospitals were not entitled to the same privileges as paying patients in the outside world, such as the right to choose their own physician.[72] And obstreperous patients clearly got short shrift, as this example from the Newcastle Infirmary suggests[73]:

> In May, 1754, a complaint as to the meat and beer was judged to be unfounded. The complaining patients were severely reprimanded, and ordered to have toast and water for a week.

Second, patients were expected to do their share in the domestic running of the hospital, so far as was compatible with their condition. For example, a resolution at the Leicester Infirmary in 1800 stated that 'such patients as are able, shall be employed in nursing the other patients, washing and ironing the linen', etc.[74]

Third, patients were to submit to moral and religious improvement. As a 1747 report of the Northampton Infirmary boldly states[75]:

> That the benefit of a Reformatory may as far as possible be added to those of an infirmary. The clergy of Northampton attended in their turn to visit the sick, to read prayers in the wards and to give communion at the proper times, for which purpose a Chalice and paten have been presented to the Society by an unknown benefactor and care is taken that the patients of all persuasions may be attended in the manner they desire.

To this end, another valued form of donation to the hospital were Bibles and other improving literature. The new wards at the Devon and Exeter, for example, were provided with 'three Bibles, three Common Prayer Books and three Books of the Whole Duty of Man',[76] while the Leicester Royal Infirmary took no fewer than 200 copies of Dr James

Stonhouse's *Friendly Advice to a Patient* and his *Spiritual Directions to the Uninstructed*.[77]

Lastly, patients who were relieved or who recovered were expected to make a public show of gratitude. Often the mode of this display was specified. At the Norfolk and Norwich for example the rule was[78]:

> that those patients discharged who have received important cures, be directed by the Chairman of the weekly Board to return public thanks at their respective places of worship, and that in any extraordinary cure the nature of the case, when proper, may be specified

and in a similar vein in Newcastle[79]:

> That when patients are discharged cured, they shall be strictly enjoined by the Chairman of the Committee, to return thanks to Almighty God in their respective places of worship and to the subscribers who recommended them.

As suggested already, the one thing the patient was not to do was to pay for his treatment. The Northampton Infirmary specified in bold type[80]:

> **HERE ARE NOW ADMITTED THE POOR, SICK LAME** (being recommended according to the rules following) and supplied with advice, medicine, diet, washing and lodging, **AND NO MONEY GIFT OR REWARD** is taken of them or their friends on any account whatever.

For monetary payment would instantly have thrown the delicate boundaries between donor and donee into utter confusion, sullied grace with commerce, and destroyed the ritual of the gift relation upon which the whole superstructure depended.

But what did all this mean in the concrete case? Did the hospitalized sick enact their prescribed roles? What was the patient's point of view? Alas, I know of no account, in any Georgian diary, autobiography, or series of letters, recording in the first person what patients actually made of their experiences of the hospital and its philanthropic scenarios. We do, however, have the next best thing, a sixty-page poem in blank verse dramatizing such experiences, written and published, by a travelling comic actor, Joseph Wilde, who spent nine weeks in the Devon and Exeter Hospital at the beginning of the nineteenth century with some kind of unspecified leg complaint.[81] Wilde's account reads as panegyric, and it presents severe interpretative problems if we try to sift fact from stereotypes served up for public consumption. Arguably, however, Wilde's text is peculiarly revealing precisely because, as an actor, he knew just how to act out the part of the grateful recipient of philanthropy within that ritual institution.

Wilde's poem reveals many details of incidental interest which illuminate the order of the Georgian infirmary. We see him, first of all, failing to gain admission at all because of the lack of a letter of recommendation (a friendly parish clerk overcomes that problem).[82] We see the medical staff visiting the wards at fixed hours each day, attended, be it noted, by a train of medical students who are their pupils.[83] We see regular visiting hours for the sufferers' friends,[84] and we see the convalescent patients expected to clean the wards, serve food, mix medicines, and generally to minister to the needs of the bedridden and the seriously sick[85]:

> Now all arise, whose ills will let them rise;
> And now, the sound of crutches and of staves
> Is heard through all the ward; but not to sloth,
> Or listless sauntering as they uprose;
> All who can wield an instrument of labour
> Are busily employ'd in cleanliness;
> Till the whole ward, for neatness, might compare,
> And wholesome sweetness, with a monarch's palace.

But, above all, perhaps, we see – because this is what Wilde dwells upon – the emotional economy of the infirmary. This has four elements. First there is Wilde's virulent antipathy to the nursing staff, scourges and scolds, unfeeling and ungracious women who for him are the veritable embodiment of uncharitable behaviour.[86] The Devon and Exeter has a complaints procedure, and Wilde records that he registered his protests against the unfeeling, uncaring nurses before that panel[87]:

'See yon poor wretch, o'erwhelm'd by dire disease,
'And long experience of the world's indifference,
'Or worse, its cruelty – his last resource
'Is in this mansion – here he hopes to find,
'At least, alleviation of his woes:
'He knows his gen'rous patrons have provided
'One of the gentler sex, in ev'ry ward,
'To be his more immediate consolation:
'How great his disappointment and dismay,
'When, for the comfort which he hop'd to meet,
'He finds, or thinks he finds, the world all bad!
'Alike inimical to poverty!
'Then sinks life's wav'ring balance, hope expires –
'Struck to the heart – he dies in deep despair.'

He doesn't report on the outcome.

Second, Wilde praises the patient community itself for its generous fund of warmth, sympathy, and kindness ('Delightful picture of humanity').[88] He presents a glowing portrait of patient mutual support, both tangible and moral, and clearly believed the psychological boost given by shared humour and cheerfulness amongst the community had great therapeutic importance[89]:

Design'd by Providence for social bliss,
The mind of man, how wonderfully fram'd,
And fitted to enjoy this feast of nature!
If for a few short days, together pent
In the same vehicle, souls sometimes mix
With souls, till both are quite averse to part;
How much more closely drawn did Thespis feel
This mortal tie, for nine long weeks immur'd
In one apartment, not a moment absent
From these his dear companions in affliction.

Join'd in one common mis'ry, grief attracts
By stronger bonds than pleasure ever knew;
The bonds of pity! What though diff'rent far
The scenes each diff'rent man is doom'd to act;
The play of life is still the same to all,
And still the same its most essential duties;
The same its natural wants, the same its end.

Fill'd with these genuine, best of human feelings,
This wide philanthropy, embracing all,
His heart expanding rises to his lips,
And thus, in tender accents, he bespeaks them:

'My dear companions, partners in mischance,
'Brothers by nature, by afflictions friends,
'And dearer grown by mutual acts of kindness,
'Full many a day, together we have past
'In friendly intercourse, not uninstructive;
'Where I've endeavour'd, and I hope not vainly,
'To merit and to gain your approbation.
'Your kind assistance in my weak condition,
'Has often fill'd my heart with gratitude;
'And such return as I had pow'r to make
'I still have made, and made it cheerfully.
'My hands, my eyes, my thoughts have been employ'd
'To aid your correspondence with your friends,
'T' explain to them your wants and speak your love:
'I know your kind concern will follow me,
'And earnest prayers for my restoration.'

Third, Wilde was positively glowing about the physicians.
His poem presents them as punctual, tactful, attentive,
finding time for cheery words to all their sufferers, and
respectful towards the battered feelings of the sick. Dr Patch
was, he says, a 'sage', but still more, he was a man. Wilde
recalls Patch's verdict on him[90]:

'Beyond all surgery' – for pity then,
The skilful doctor for awhile was lost
In the more noble character – the man:
And though inur'd to sights of deepest woe,
The starting tear proclaim'd the feeling heart:
This tribute paid to sweet Humanity.

Clearly, to judge from Wilde's account, the medical staff
perfectly acted out their role as benevolent dispensers of
science and sympathy.

And, last, Wilde had nothing but praise for the hospital
itself ('blest institution'),[91] both in its objects and their
execution. Indeed he dedicated his work to its supporters.

There is not a hint in his lines of the reservations and second thoughts about the efficacy of infirmaries one finds expressed by John Aikin, or, somewhat later, by Thomas Beddoes.[92] For Wilde, no praise was too high for the humanity of the subscribers; and gratitude duly poured from his lips.[93]

'When I reflect on all I have beheld,
'On all I have experienc'd in this mansion,
'When I survey the heart-affecting sight,
'Which now presents itself before mine eyes,
'These, the restor'd, and you their blest restorers,
'My heart, o'erwhelm'd, becomes too full for praise;
'And praise, if I could utter, were presumptuous,
'Where thanks and blessings only should be pour'd.
'That I am thankful for the kindness shewn me,
'Witness these tears which flow not now for grief,
'Or disappointment at my loss of hope:
'My heart has long been satisfy'd in this,
''Tis not in Science to avert my fate,
'Else had I found my restoration here.'

At one level, of course, the hospital gift relation was nothing other than traditional paternalism institutionalized, the stewardship of the rich towards the poor, humanitarian but ultimately conservative. But also, in a slightly more refined sense, the voluntary hospital represented a subtle device whereby the governing classes could enjoy the advantages of treating most of the poor most of the time through the repressive policing mechanisms of the poor law, while also being able personally to lend their names to more prestigious institutions for handpicked members of the labouring classes, institutions of which they could be visibly proud, and which put an idealized gloss upon their relations with the poor. And at the same time the voluntary hospital represents the classic medium through which, by joint subscription action, the polite and propertied initiated their own act of national renewal, meeting through association, philanthropy, and culture new social challenges, which could no longer be met by the established institutions of old corruption. It is a measure of the satisfactoriness – to the donors – of all those moves that the voluntary hospital system lasted with minimal alterations for no less than two centuries.

Notes

1. Laurence Sterne, *A Sentimental Journey*, ed. by G Petrie (Penguin Books, Harmondsworth, 1982), 31.

2. Quoted in David Owen, *English Philanthropy 1660–1960* (Cambridge, Mass., Belknap Press, 1965), 11; see also Donna Andrew, 'London charity in the eighteenth century' (PhD thesis, University of Toronto, 1977).

3. See Owen, *English Philanthropy*, note 2.

4. J. Aikin, *Thoughts on Hospitals* (London, Johnson, 1771).

5. See J. Woodward, *To Do the Sick No Harm: A Study of the British Voluntary Hospital System to 1875* (London, Routledge & Kegan Paul, 1974); F.N.L. Poynter (ed.), *The Evolution of Hospitals in Britain* (London, Pitman, 1968); S.G. Cherry, 'The role of the English provincial hospitals in the 18th and 19th centuries' (PhD thesis, University of East Anglia, 1977); W.H. McMenemey, 'The hospital movement of the eighteenth century and its development', in Poynter, *The Evolution of Hospitals in Britain*, 43–72. Note that the present essay confines itself to English provincial hospitals. Nothing is said about either London or Scotland. Nor is it intended to be a general survey of the functions fulfilled by the voluntary hospital.

6. Quoted in Owen, *English Philanthropy*, 14. See also Alured Clarke, *A Sermon preached in the Cathedral Church of Winchester before the Governors of the County Hospital at the opening on October 18th 1736*, Winchester, and *A Sermon preached before the Trustees of the Charity Schools at the Cathedral Church of Exeter on 13th October 1741*, Exeter.

7. H. Bevan, *Records of the Salop Infirmary* (Shrewsbury, by order of the Board of Directors, 1847), 6.

8. R.M. Clay, *The Medieval Hospitals of England* (London, Methuen, 1909).

9. Alexander Pope, *Essay on Man*, epistle III.

10. E.P. Thompson, *Whigs and Hunters* (London, Allen Lane, 1957); D. Hay, P. Linebaugh and E.P. Thompson (eds) *Albion's Fatal Tree* (London, Allen Lane, 1975).

11. Betsy Rodgers, *Cloak of Charity. Studies in Eighteenth Century Philanthropy* (London, Methuen, 1949).

12. I. Maddox, *The Duty and Advantages of Encouraging Public Infirmaries*, 3rd edn (London, J. Brotherton, 1743), 6.

13. Maddox, *Duty and Advantages*, 17. Maddox writes:

> The various apprehensions of mankind, the different opinions entertained upon points of government and policy, as well as upon subjects of a higher nature, are too often apt to inflame the passions, create animosities, and produce, at best, a cold disregard; sometimes, it is to be feared, much rage and fierceness: but this mutual intercourse in works of charity, smooths and rubs off these asperities. A joint labour of love,

by uniting in some measure the views of different persons, forms a kind of friendly cement; softens the angry passions, and abates that severe and harsh opinion, which men of disagreeing sentiments and views are too ready to entertain and propagate upon the whole character of one another.

14. Geoffrey Holmes and W.A. Speck, *The Divided Society. Party Conflict in England 1694–1716* (London, Edward Arnold, 1967).

15. E.R. Frizelle and J.D. Martin, *The Leicester Royal Infirmary 1771–1971* (Leicester, Leicester No. 1 Hospital Management Committee, 1971), 26.

16. J.D. Harris, *The Royal Devon and Exeter Hospital* (Exeter, Eland, 1922),16.

17. J. Priestley, *A Sermon On Behalf of the Leeds Infirmary preached at Mill Hill Chapel* . . . (Leek, 1768), 19.

18. F.F. Waddy, *A History of Northampton General Hospital 1743 to 1948* (Northampton, Guildhall Press, 1974). See also Philip Doddridge, 'Compassion to the sick recommended and urged', in Job Orton (ed.), *The Works of Philip Doddridge, D.D.*, vol. iv (London, 1804).

19. J.D. Harris, *The Royal Devon and Exeter Hospital*, 13.

20. G. Munro-Smith, *A History of the Bristol Royal Infirmary* (Bristol and London, Arrowsmith, 1917). See also Jonathan Barry, 'The cultural life of Bristol, 1640–1775' (DPhil thesis, University of Oxford, 1985).

21. Frizelle and Martin, *The Leicester Royal Infirmary*, 27.

22. P.M.G. Russell, *A History of the Exeter Hospitals, 1170–1948* (Exeter, Exeter Medical Post-Graduate Institute, 1976).

23. Munro-Smith, *Bristol Royal Infirmary*, 37.

24. J.V. Pickstone and S.V.F. Butler, 'The politics of medicine in Manchester, 1788–1792: hospital reform and public health services in the early industrial city', *Medical History*, 28 (1984), 227–49; W. Brockbank, *Portrait of a Hospital 1752–1948* (London, Heinemann, 1952); John V. Pickstone, *Medicine and Industrial Society. A History of Hospital Development in Manchester and its Region, 1752–1946* (Manchester, Manchester University Press, 1985), 10ff., and, for nineteenth-century charities, 42–62.

25. For conceptual background see R.H. Titmuss, *The Gift Relationship* (London, George Allen & Unwin, 1970).

26. See W.F. Bynum, 'Health, disease and medical care', in G.S. Rousseau and Roy Porter (eds), *The Ferment of Knowledge* (Cambridge, Cambridge University Press, 1980), 211–54.

27. For discussion of that culture see P.J. Corfield, *The Impact of English Towns, 1700–1800* (Oxford, Oxford University Press, 1982).

28. See G.H. Hume, *The History of the Newcastle Infirmary* (Newcastle-upon-Tyne, Andrew Reid & Co., 1906).

29. Carole Rawcliffe, 'The hospitals of later medieval London', *Medical History*, 28 (1984), 1–21.

30. Sir Humphry Rolleston, *The Cambridge Medical School* (Cambridge, Cambridge University Press, 1932).

31. Priestley, *A Sermon*, 11.

32. Bevan, *Salop Infirmary*, 6.

33. J. Money, *Experience and Identity. Birmingham and the West Midlands 1760–1800* (Manchester, Manchester University Press, 1977), 84; see also Frizelle and Martin, *Leicester Royal Infirmary*, 74–5.

34. J. Latimer, *The Annals of Bristol in the Eighteenth Century* (reprinted, Bath, Kingsmead Reprints, 1970), ii, 318.

35. Waddy, *Northampton General Hospital*, 6.

36. J.D. Leader and S. Snell, *Sheffield Royal Infirmary, 1797–1897* (Sheffield, Sheffield Infirmary, 1897), 6.

37. Owen, *English Philanthropy*, 12–13.

38. Sir P. Eade, *The Norfolk and Norwich Hospital 1779–1900* (London, Jarrold, 1900), 17. See also E. Copeman, *Brief History of the Norfolk and Norwich Hospital* (Norwich, 1856).

39. G. Whitcombe, *The General Infirmary at Gloucester* (Gloucester, John Bellows, 1903), 9.

40. Eade, *Norfolk and Norwich Hospital*, 36.

41. F.H. Jacob, *A History of the General Hospital near Nottingham* (Bristol and London, Wright, 1951), 16. For the same at Northampton, see Waddy, *Northampton General Hospital*, 5.

42. Sir F. Hill, *Georgian Lincoln* (Cambridge, Cambridge University Press, 1966), 71. See also T. Sympson, *A Short Account of the Old and of the New Lincoln County Hospitals* (London, J. Williamson, 1878). The genteel nature of such hospitals is emphasized in Charles Webster, 'The crisis of the hospitals during the industrial revolution', in E. Forbes (ed.), *Human Implications of Scientific Advance* (Edinburgh, Edinburgh University Press, 1978), 214–23.

43. Salisbury General Hospital, *Salisbury 200 – The Bicentenary of Salisbury Infirmary, 1766-1966* (Salisbury, Salisbury General Hospital, 1967), 15.

44. Jacob, *Nottingham General Hospital*, 25.

45. C.T. Andrews, *The First Cornish Hospital* (Truro, the author, 1975).

46. Leader and Snell, *Sheffield Royal Infirmary*, 12; for the parallel at Nottingham, see Jacob, *Nottingham General Hospital*, title page.

47. David Cannadine, *Lords and Landlords. The Aristocracy and the Towns, 1774–1967* (Leicester, Leicester University Press, 1980).

48. See Money, *Experience and Identity*; see also C. Pye, *A Brief Account of the General Hospital near Birmingham* (Birmingham, 1820); J.M. Hall and V.C. Harral, *The General Hospital, Birmingham* (Birmingham, University of Birmingham Hospital, 1967). For Yorkshire see H.H. Marland, *Medicine and Society in Wakefield and Huddersfield 1780–1870* (Cambridge, Cambridge University Press, 1987).

49. Russell, *Exeter Hospitals*, 26.

50. Geoffrey Holmes, *Augustan England, Professions, State and Society*

1680–1730 (London, George Allen & Unwin, 1982); I. Loudon, 'The nature of provincial medical practice in eighteenth century England', *Medical History*, 29 (1985), 1–32.

51. W.H. McMenemey, *A History of the Worcester Royal Infirmary* (Worcester and London, Press Alliances, 1947), 20.

52. Rodgers, *Cloak of Charity*, 7.

53. Maddox, *Duty and Advantages*, 24.

54. Rodgers, *Cloak of Charity*, 8; Owen, *English Philanthropy*, 14.

55. J.T. Anning, *The General Infirmary at Leeds*, vol. 1, *The First Hundred Years* (Edinburgh, E. & S. Livingstone, 1963), 1.

56. Priestley, *A Sermon*, 10.

57. Frizelle and Martin, *Leicester Royal Infirmary*, 24. Watts continued:

Herein public and private good are most intimately combined. Herein we are called to be charitable in an age, and nation, and instance, in which Charity superabounds. These inducements therefore it is to be hoped accompanied with that inward Testimony which cannot but arise in every compassionate breast, will effectually actuate all, each according to their circumstances and degree, to prove themselves truly friends to the poor, to the county, to the kingdom, to mankind. In *this*, and every other humane, polite, charitable, and christian, regard, may the very respectable county of Leicester ever, under the divine influence, be an example and praise to this land of Liberty and social Virtue: This land of Liberty and social Virtue ever, under the divine Influence, be an example, and praise, to the whole Earth!

58. Owen, *English Philanthropy*, 38.

59. Priestley, *A Sermon*, 10.

60. Waddy, *Northampton General Hospital*, 6.

61. Owen, *English Philanthropy*, 38.

62. Jacob, *Nottingham General Hospital*, 18. Compare the same argument used by the advocates of the Leicester Infirmary:

Whereas many sick and lame persons languish (deprived even of the due Necessaries of Life at a time when more particularly required) and too often die miserably partly for want of Accommodations and proper Medicines in their own Houses or Lodgings, and partly by the inprudent laying out of the small Pittance allowed by their Parishes and by the Ignorance or ill Management of those about them, thro' which they suffer extreamly, nay are sometimes lost. (Frizelle and Martin, *Leicester Royal Infirmary*, 33.

63. See Woodward, *To Do the Sick No Harm*, 14.

64. Priestley, *A Sermon*, 18.

65. W.S. Lewis and R.M. Williams, *Private Charity in England 1747–1757* (New Haven, Yale University Press, 1938).

66. Maddox, *Duty and Advantages*, 3.

67. W.B. Howie, 'The administration of an eighteenth century provincial hospital', *Medical History*, 5 (1961), 34–55, 50. For a European perspective on the population of eighteenth-century hospitals, see A. Imhof, 'The hospital in the eighteenth century: for whom?', *Journal of Social History*, 10 (1970), 448–70. For Scotland see Guenter Risse, *Hospital Life in Enlightenment Scotland* (Cambridge, Cambridge University Press, 1986), especially Chs 1 and 2.

68. Howie, 'Administration', 37.

69. Eade, *Norfolk and Norwich Hospital*, 56.

70. Priestley, *A Sermon*, 18.

71. Howie, 'Administration', 52.

72. T. Percival, *Medical Ethics* (Manchester, J. Jackson, 1803).

73. Hume, *Newcastle Infirmary*, 25.

74. Frizelle and Martin, *Leicester Royal Infirmary*, 58. Howie, 'Administration', records the following (53):

In 1786 the Nurse in the Male Ward complained to the Weekly Board of Thomas Virnall, a patient in the Ward 'for refusing to give her the customary assistance in fomenting such Patients as are not able to do it for themselves.' He pled in his defence 'that his hands were so very tender that he could not bear the operation'. He was reprimanded. (*Minutes*, 17 July 1786)

75. Waddy, *Northampton General Hospital*, 9.

76. Harris, *Devon and Exeter Hospital*, 29.

77. Frizelle and Martin, *Leicester Royal Infirmary*, 60. See also J. Stonhouse, *Friendly Advice to a Patient*, 9th ed. (London, J. Rivington, 1750).

78. Eade, *Norfolk and Norwich Hospital*, 61.

79. Hume, *Newcastle Infirmary*, 11.

80. Waddy, *Northampton General Hospital*, 6.

81. Joseph Wilde, *The Hospital, a Poem in Three Books, Written in the Devon and Exeter Hospital, 1809* (Norwich, Stevenson, Matchett, and Stevenson, 1809). See W.B. Howie, 'Consumer reaction: a patient's view of hospital life in 1809', *British Medical Journal*, 3 (1973), 534–6.

82. Wilde, *The Hospital*, 6–7.

83. Op. cit., 17.

84. Op. cit., 42.

85. Op. cit., 27, 31.

86. Op. cit., 56.

87. Op. cit., 58.

88. Op. cit., 29.

89. Op. cit., 61–3.

90. Op. cit., 18.

91. Op. cit., 55.

92. John Aikin, *Thoughts on Hospitals* (London, Johnson, 1771); J.E. Stock, *Memoir of the Life of Thomas Beddoes, M.D.* (London, J. Murray, 1811), appendix 3, 'Considerations on infirmaries'.

93. Wilde, *Hospital*, 67.

III

Modern

7

An historical survey of children's hospitals[1]

Eduard Seidler

The development of the children's hospital has received systematic appraisal from neither historians of pediatrics nor historians of medicine and medical institutions. In particular, we lack any in-depth studies on the motives which have spurred both medicine and wider society to establish this distinctive institution.

This paper does not pretend to compensate in any comprehensive manner for this gap in the literature, but it does hope at least to draw attention to a number of elements peculiar to the history of the children's hospital and worthy of more detailed study. Speaking from the standpoint of a pediatrician, all too conscious of the problems plaguing the concept of the children's hospital today, my strategy here is not to construct some abstract chronology, but to attempt a critical overview of the various approaches people under different historical circumstances have adopted to the problem of the children's hospital. The question at hand cannot be formulated simply enough: What leads people to establish institutions for sick children, what form do these institutions take, and what is their function understood to be?

The child in hospital

The children's hospital has its roots in the eighteenth century's radical transformation of the old 'hospital' – home of refuge, into the '*Krankenhaus*' – institution for the care of the sick. Before the eighteenth century, it would not be correct to call any institution of the Christian social service system a 'hospital' as we understand the term today. It cannot be stressed enough that the setting up of homes of refuge for pilgrims, misfits, the poor, the lame – and also certain groups of children – must be understood in the context of a Christian culture dedicated to the protection of the helpless. As such, the old hospital was not, or only incidentally, concerned with special care for the ill. In principle, it was still the same institution for the poor and needy which the council fathers in Nicaea had established when, in the year 375 AD, they made it the duty of every diocese to address itself to the physical, mental, and social sufferings of its flock. This old concept of the hospital, while manifesting itself institutionally in a variety of forms over the succeeding centuries, never ceased to be strictly an organization for the care and refuge of the poor and sick; it was never conceived as an institution of medicine. It belonged, rather, to the Church, the lay sisters, and later the towns, the princes, or the state.

If we look for children in this hospital system, we find the unwanted, the abandoned, the orphaned, but hardly any truly sick children. This is not the place to involve ourselves in the complex history of foundling hospitals and orphanages, in which this hospital system certainly played a role. It will suffice at this juncture simply to note that, as long as an extremely high rate of child mortality was tolerated by society, so long as the long-term survival of every newborn child was not perceived as part of the medical profession's responsibilities, as long as the state also saw no reason to look upon child mortality as a problem with which it should concern itself, then it was left to humanitarian and charity groups to take on a child if its parents – for whatever reason – were no longer able or willing to care for it. To just what extent, then, the history of the children's hospital can be simply understood in the broad context of social history, and how far it touches on the deeper biosocial problem of human ambivalence towards the weakness and absolute dependence of the child, can here only be posed as a question.[2]

Before the eighteenth century, our knowledge of everyday life, including the everyday life of the sick or helpless child, whether at home or in a hospital, is so meagre that it is impossible to make any sort of authoritative statement. We know though, if only sketchily, that coexisting with the special foundling hospitals and orphanages, there were apparently nurseries in many general hospitals. This was especially true of the larger hospitals, such as the Hôtel-Dieu in Paris, St Bartholomew's in London, Heilig-Geist in Nürnberg, Juliusspital in Würzburg, just to mention a few. These nurseries, however, simply acted as an additional component of a complex network of social services for the poor and needy; they were not specially conceived as medical units, i.e. as special institutions for the care of sick children.

All this began to change only in the time of the European Enlightenment, when the child as a concept, as a social entity, began to take on a new significance. Briefly put, we are concerned in this period with a society which, caught in the throes of a growing sense of nationalistic sentiment, no longer looked upon the child as a poor weak wretch who might as well die as live, but which increasingly celebrated its children as the bearers of its hopes for the future; and which consequently came to see the survival and healthy development of its children as the only guarantee of its own continuing existence. The imperative of national survival, then, implied that the medical profession (working with the schoolteachers) was duty bound to help the vulnerable child raise itself to a level of physical integrity and intellectual independence sufficient to allow it ultimately to take its place in society as a responsible adult.

The change from hospital to *Krankenhaus*

In the eighteenth and early nineteenth centuries, the medical profession took it upon itself to reorganize the old hospitals in three ways. Where previously doctors had visited these institutions only occasionally as consultants, now these hospitals were increasingly used:

1 as centres for medical training;
2 as clinical laboratories for medical research – a development with especially wide-reaching consequences; and
3 finally, though rather later, as an organization of healing concerned with the welfare of the population.

All these developments were part and parcel of a more general splintering and reorganization of the old hospital of refuge and care into a conglomerate of new specialized institutions of social welfare, one of these being medical. The *Krankenhaus*, with its broad aim of admitting and healing sick persons, thus came into being, along with a wide range of other new social institutions, asylums, and homes. Under the influence of the *égalité* of the French Revolution, moreover, these new institutions aimed, at least in principle, to extend their services to every citizen.[3]

For sick children, two competing systems of care and treatment were offered, the modern-day descendants of which have remained in conflict to the present day.

1 Outpatient care, or care for the child by the medical profession which allows it to remain in its own familiar surroundings at home.
2 Inpatient care, which takes the sick child into a special institution with the aim of re-establishing its health before returning it to its family.

Three well-known historical examples will allow us to see the concrete working-out of this two-pronged system. The first *ambulatorium*, or outpatient dispensary for sick children, established in 1769 by George Armstrong in London (7 Red Lion Square), normally receives merely glancing attention from historians of pediatrics, especially since it was forced to close in 1782 for 'lack of public interest and support'.[4] Yet this institution's conceptual importance earns it a key place in the history of the children's hospital, since it established the basic idea that sick children require a type of institutionalized care distinct from that called for in the case of adults.

'To administer advice and medicines gratis to the children of the Industrious Poor, from the birth to the age of 10 or 12 years' – this was the high ideal of this new dispensary, which Armstrong saw as 'charity of the greatest consequence to the Public'.[5] Not the increase of medical knowledge, but the saving of 'a great many lives very useful to the Public' was the aim. Among an intellectual elite, keen to maintain the more mundane cogs of their comfortable society in good working order, the Armstrong dispensary was conceived as a 'nursery for labourers, tradesmen, soldiers, and sailors'. A proud figure of nearly 35,000 children – or about eight children per day – treated by Armstrong's unit between 1769 and 1781, speaks volumes for the success of the experiment:

> As persons in the lower stations of life have a more free intercourse and communication with one another, than those of a higher rank, and make their children a more frequent topic of conversation, for want of other subjects, and being also less liable to dissipation, it is natural to imagine, that by means of this charity the above mentioned instructions are now become generally known and observed by the Industrious Poor in and about London.[6]

After Armstrong's institution was forced to close its doors, one sees, both in England and on the continent, a number of further attempts – today mostly forgotten – to develop the idea of the dispensary as an ideal institutional model for the medical treatment of sick children. The Royal Infirmary for Children, founded in London in 1816 by Davis, had three departments in the city and was almost entirely devoted to the treatment of outpatients. On the other hand, in 1852 when Charles West in Great Ormond Street in London, began to realize his long-cherished wish for a real children's hospital, this was no further development of the Armstrong 'social-pediatric' dispensary, but was an expression of the larger attempt of the time to raise English institutions to the standard of scientific excellence represented by the Paris and Vienna schools of clinical pathology.[7]

Meanwhile, on the continent, Joseph Johann Mastalier's *Kinderkrankeninstitut* had emerged in 1788 as an expression of the philanthropic impulses of an enlightened Viennese absolutism, with much family resemblance to the (now-defunct) British dispensary of Armstrong.[8] In a petition to the Emperor dated 1792, the order of priority of Mastalier's concerns was clearly delineated. At the top of the list was the 'charitable act' of providing children 'with necessary aid in the simplest, swiftest manner, and involving the minimum of costs'. Ranking second was the issue of wider social benefit; it was clear that the nation as a whole would 'profit greatly' if its mothers were better informed on the rules for healthy living. Finally – and clearly of lesser significance – it was noted that the new institute would offer 'an important advantage for the medical sciences', allowing them the opportunity to make 'some useful discoveries' through 'closer observation of children's illnesses'. In contrast to the London experiment, Mastalier's small institution proved itself robust; out of its humble beginnings emerged, under Leopold Anton Gölis, the 'first public children's hospital' in Vienna. This institution, however, was finally completed only in 1837 by Ludwig Wilhhelm Mauthner, who had been prodded into action by the founding of the first children's hospitals in Germany and Austria.

I have chosen to focus on these two small institutions because they are illustrative of one type of child medical care which would continue to find form throughout the later history of the children's hospital. The underprivileged ('deserving poor') child represented the first object of structured pediatrics. Only much later, as we well know, would the general outpatient clinics, concerned all along with children and the poor, spawn their specialized pediatric facilities and children's clinics. Indeed, much of what is said today about 'social pediatrics' as a supposedly new dimension of child medical care, was – from prevention to aftercare – clearly anticipated in these early pediatric institutions.

At this point, it is necessary to take a closer look at those two institutional 'types' with which the true children's hospital would most intimately come to identify, and whose beginnings are to be found at the Hôpital des Enfants Malades at the Rue de Sèvres in Paris.

The history of this institution, so pertinent to our problem, has unfortunately hardly been investigated. The brief official canons tell the proud story of how the decree of the 9th Floréal of the tenth year of the Revolution (29 April 1802) effected the transformation of the orphanage Maison de l'Enfant Jésus into the first children's hospital in the world.

As might be expected, the real situation was much more complex, emerging in the first instance more as an administrative and social drama than a medical one.[9] In France, since the Renaissance, since the days of François I and Vincent de Paul, it had been widely agreed that children had no business in hospitals and other institutions designed for adults. The fact that they were in fact sent to such places was repeatedly denounced as a scandal and a disgrace. Among the widely discussed reports was one from the Hôtel-Dieu, where not only in the nursery, but also in the adult wards, up to eight children were forced to share one bed – with over 90 per cent becoming prey to certain death as a result of infection. The famous, and for hospital history so important, memorial written by Jacques René Tenon in 1788 strongly argued for at least equipping the new hospitals with special wards for children under 12 years old.[10]

By setting aside 250 beds for children under 15 in a large building 'vaste, aéré et propre', the new hospital hoped to achieve three things: first, to set up a precise line of demarcation between the adults and children; second, to put itself in a position to achieve a more precise classification of the children according to illness; and third, to encourage the ethically-desirable possibility of discharging the children less 'corrumpus' than had been the case when they were mixed indiscriminately in with the adults in general hospitals.

For some time, then, we hear nothing about a children's hospital based on a medical conception, if we disregard the fact that only acutely ill children were to be admitted to the new hospital, while those with infectious diseases and the chronically ill were to be taken to the Hôpital des Vénériens or the Hôpital Saint-Louis.

The large Parisian clinics, which arose during the post-Revolutionary years, e.g. by converting large monastery buildings, aimed to provide the increasingly prestigious clinical/pathological Paris School with new scientific knowledge and facts.[11] The large number of patients and conveniently high mortality rate offered French doctors the opportunity of perfecting their clinical-anatomical localizationist approach to illness and its treatment, which had been steadily gaining adherents since the days of Morgagni. Paris became the centre of this revolution in medical methodology, with men such as Corvisart, Laënnec, Bichat, and Broussais paving the way for later workers.

The pediatric institution at Rue de Sèvres established itself in this school soon after its foundation. In fact, fundamental scientific research into children's diseases based on the new methods began here. Soon it was almost exclusively oriented towards the gaining of knowledge for medical science, with comparatively little concern for the care of the afflicted.

Pediatrics is indebted to these efforts to correlate the first complete descriptions of children's illnesses with pathological/anatomical findings. The impact of this pioneering work continues to make itself felt in nosology up to the present day. It should be said, however, that even while doctors of the time prided themselves on their advanced research methods, a basic rationale for the founding of the Hôpital des Enfants Malades, i.e. systematic separation of the children from one another according to illness, was completely forgotten. Up to the end of the century people complained of hospital epidemics; however, for the enterprising physicians these were an object of scientific interest no less than the range of primary diseases. 'One has,' the famous Tübingen clinician Carl August Wunderlich wrote home in 1841, 'ample opportunity to study especially infectious diseases, which do not die out even after all possible measures of containment are applied'.[12] Even today we have very little information about this hospital, described later by Rauchfuss as an 'excellent organisation of *traitement externe*'.[13] These words of praise can be put into perspective by noting that this outpatient treatment mentioned by Rauchfuss apparently played only a minor role in the functioning of the institution as a whole.

I have deliberately discussed the background of the founding of these institutions of child medical care in considerable detail because I believe we cannot discuss such institutions as abstract isolated historical curiosities, but must attempt to integrate them into the constitutional structure of the children's hospital as a concept. Back in the nineteenth century, Franz Seraphim Hügel had already identified the three types: the *Kinderkrankeninstitute*, the *Kinderkrankenhäuser*, and the *Kinderbewahrungsinstitute*, thereby specifying that children might either be visited at home, admitted to an institution as outpatients and given specific treatment, or taken out of their family environment into care.[14]

Up to this point, we have seen that different institutions were established to deal with all these tasks. Whereas all forms of day nurseries were seen as 'sickness/palliative institutions', the institutes for children's diseases were concerned with outpatient consultation and home visits. Over time, the children's hospital, conceived for the purpose of diagnosing and treating sick children, came to dominate these other institutions, largely as a result of its association with pediatric research. Unfortunately, it did not take long before the dangers as well as the opportunities afforded by this development made themselves felt, notably in the pernicious phenomenon which would come to be known worldwide as 'hospitalism'.

Structural elements of the children's hospital

In 1877, the German-Russian pediatrician Carl Rauchfuss presented his detailed analysis of the children's hospital in the first international *Handbuch der Kinderkrankheiten*.[15] By this time, so many individual examples of the institution had arisen internationally that he could venture to construct what, to his mind, would represent the optimal model.

> If one were simply to build children's hospitals along exactly the same construction and with the same furnishing, equipment and organization as the general hospitals, then it would not be worthwhile building them at all; it would then be advisable to recognise the appropriateness of expanding on the practice of many already established general hospitals of treating sick children in a children's ward. The requirements of a children's hospital are, however, more complicated than those of a general hospital, and these incorporated children's wards are compelled under the circumstances to do without.[16]

Rauchfuss, who here unremittingly propagated the model for an independent children's hospital, wanted to unite all elements of child care under one roof. With a capacity of ten beds and 500 outpatients per 10,000 inhabitants, he believed it would be possible to cope, providing the following structural elements were established:

1 An outpatients' department, separate from that of the inpatients. The main advantage of such a department 'is self-evident', meriting the greatest attention and interest from all involved. Rauchfuss stressed, however, that it should not be serviced by already exhausted physicians

from the inpatient department.

2 An observation or quarantine ward, connected to each of the different main wards.

3 Isolation houses serving, if possible, every conceivable form of illness, including mixed cases.

4 Play and gymnastic halls, rooms for physiotherapy, and garden areas.

Reactions to Rauchfuss's proposals instructively highlight the massive objections to which the concept of the children's hospital at this time was susceptible. The high rates of infection and mortality within these institutions had raised the question, not only among the general population but in the medical world as well, as to whether children's hospitals deserved to exist at all. A more subtle objection had been raised by Florence Nightingale, who – exploiting the full weight of her authority – had made the case that children collectively were incapable of mature analysis and assessment, and so their complaints could not be taken into consideration as a guideline for assessing the care they required. Without such a feedback from the charges, however, it would be difficult to run a hospital efficiently. These considerations led Nightingale to recommend that sick children be put alongside the adults once more, preferably in the women's wards.[17]

The main problem, though, was and remained that of infection, a fact which led Rauchfuss and his generation to envisage the future of the children's hospital exclusively as a decentralized institution dedicated to 'the perfecting of the construction, furnishing, equipment and staffing' of the isolation houses.

The isolationist trend dreamt of by Rauchfuss would in fact become the favoured trend among builders of children's hospitals, as knowledge from bacteriology helped pediatric research achieve its first publicly recognized breakthrough – the decline of child mortality. The questions raised as to the value of the children's hospital increasingly had to be weighed against the plainly growing improvements in the institution's infrastructure: the introduction of cubicles, increased decentralization, measures for antisepsis and asepsis. The growing number of scientific arguments supporting all these measures not only helped relieve the hospitals of the accusation that they were little better than houses of death, but also permitted them to admit certain classes of children which had previously been treated only as outpatients or not at all, especially infants.

When Arthur Schlossmann, one of the most famous German pediatricians of his time, opened his 'Säuglingsheim' in Dresden in 1904, he had to give it this name instead of the originally intended 'Säuglings-Heilanstalt', in order to avoid the intrigue aimed against him on the grounds of unfair competition.[18] It was his belief that an

> institute run by specialists for sick infants [should] be established, which – in a fully self-contained fashion – should fulfil the special demands of infant hygiene, have its own trained nursing staff and specially trained doctors and management and, if at all possible, not be affiliated with a large hospital, but rather with an obstetric institution in order to have access to wet nurses or breast-feeding by the mother.

Not to be withheld in this connection is the fact that other pediatricians at this time were making the case for the infant hospital in candid social Darwinistic tones. The fact that more interest had been devoted to 'worthless' idiots, deaf-mutes, and cripples than to 'preventing the demise of normal human beings' was denounced as a pernicious consequence of the 'singular confusion [produced by] the emotion of humanitarianism'. Far better if society directed its philanthropic instinct to improving its system of infant care. 'If the century just begun is to become a century for the child', wrote the Aachen paediatrician J.J.G. Rey in 1906, then the first task of pediatrics lay in infant care.[19]

Yet the idea of separate infant-care institutions was not to be realized. On the contrary, the children's hospitals strived increasingly to take advantage of this new opportunity to put their capabilities to the test, either by establishing their own infant departments or by setting up day nurseries. Having taken over responsibility for infants, the children's hospital gained a new reputation for self-centredness and aloofness, and it cannot be denied that its further development was in fact increasingly inward-looking and oriented towards its own needs. The old interest in outpatient treatment declined markedly; the outpatient stations gradually turning into selective admission departments. Special departments for convalescence, for chronically sick children, and for the incurable were established. There was hardly any children's hospital which did not work in close co-operation with one or another children's sanatorium for tuberculosis, scrofula, anaemia, or rickets; or did not have its own salt-water spa, seaside hospital, or high altitude health resort. This specialization, with its useful and its problematic consequences, led in turn to something else: the operating theatres (along with their special patients) migrated from the children's clinics to newly-established special children's departments in surgical hospitals.

When the Deutsche Gesellschaft für Kinderheilkunde offered the opportunity in Hamburg in 1928 to discuss, on an international level, the problem of the children's hospital, hardly any aspect of the new infrastructure of this institution received a mention.[20] Emil Feer emphasised merely two features as relevant compared to the general hospital: first, the establishment of specially strict measures to be taken when admitting child patients with an infectious disease, in order to prevent the infection of the other patients; and, second, the establishment of special infant-care stations, milk kitchens, and a system facilitating access to wet nurses. Otherwise, the demands raised in 1928 for separate isolation departments or department houses and for the setting up of isolation wards were the same as those of fifty years previously. The only thing that strikes one's attention in this new report is that outpatient treatment is no longer specifically mentioned as a goal of the children's hospital. A planner has to decide, said Feer, whether he prefers centralization or decentralization; he himself was in favour of a series of self-contained units operating within a system of linking corridors. Finally, Feer appealed to the likely financial backers of such an institution, declaring that, after all, a good children's hospital must be able to meet the most exacting of standards, for 'the responsibility is too great for us to undertake to run a children's hospital with inadequate means and facilities'.[21]

The home for sick children

Arthur Schlossmann, whose official task it was to report on the care of children suffering from infectious diseases, chose in the 1928 meeting to swing back and strike a surprise blow by reproving the isolated hospital and its sterile historical developments – with emphasis on both senses of the word. 'The children's hospital is dead!' he cried out. 'Long live the home for sick children!'[22] To the horror of many colleagues, he demanded, in place of independent children's hospitals, large pediatric departments in general central hospitals, which he held to represent the ideal and most economic institution for public health care. The long-bemoaned problem of infection he noted, was in the present age principally under control, and matters could only improve. Thus, all individuals under the age of 14 should, with respect to 'hygiene, finance and general medical management . . . come under the supervision of the pediatrician'. Moreover – and here Schlossmann touched on a problem he considered particularly important – 'children have no business in eye clinics, ear clinics, so-called surgical tuberculosis wards, or even skin clinics; [all such child patients] belong together in children's departments'. Schlossmann was convinced 'The best care for our patients stems from cooperation with other specialists. With the integration of the children's departments into the large general hospitals, we have the possibility of ensuring the best specialist treatment and assistance at any hour.' In those cases where the internist or surgeon on his own attempts treatment, it becomes all too easy to lose sight of the fact that the individual, not the illness, is the ultimate object of medical care.

It would take us too far afield to give a report on the extremely interesting international discussion which ensued as a result of both the above-mentioned contributions and the other lectures; one can read them in the 1928 issue of the *Monatsschrift für Kinderheilkunde*. It remains only to mention the comment made during the discussion by the famous Munich pediatrician Meinhard von Pfaundler who, with his demand for a special pediatric surgeon under one's own roof, anticipated the new trend towards super-specialization familiar to us today.

Before we finally ask whether this historical overview of the development of the children's hospital has provided any useful data for helping us cope with the problems of today and tomorrow, let us briefly cast a glance at the closing main points of discussion which were given consideration at a 1957 meeting of the Deutsche Krankenhausinstitut and the pediatricians.[23] This is quickly accomplished, as we can readily ascertain that hardly any significant new issues were raised, though a great many unimportant ones insisted on making themselves heard. The problem of infection – here Schlossmann had been proved right – was no longer associated with the classical 'children's diseases', but had instead become the stigma of care for premature infants. Fanconi saw the age of single cubicles and lobbies as at an end, and argued for the establishment of four- and six-bed rooms or even wards, where the children might feel 'very happy'.[24] He went on to say that a distinction should be made between hospitals for the chronically sick, in which 'family life should be reproduced as far as possible', and hospitals for patients with acute conditions, for whom the optimal solution was a 'self-contained high-rise building', allowing the shortest possible travelling-distance from one department to another. In addition, larger children's hospitals should be built, he thought, as it was only there that recently-developed expensive specialized equipment could properly be put to use. For the same reason, a small children's hospital could only really function efficiently in liaison with a larger general hospital. As things turned out, psychological and administrative pressures on the children's hospital have led to a situation in which social customs and living standards define the parameters within which decisions and plans are made, far more than advances in medicine.

In the same discussion of 1957, in the course of an extensive survey outlining once again general operational principles for the running of a children's hospital, Joachim Wolff and Horst Sahl expressed their desire to create a 'Lebensraum' for each patient in accordance with his or her condition, age, and illness.[25] They reasoned that the children's hospital had basically to cater to the needs of four classes of patients: 'the premature infant, the baby, the toddler, and the school-age child with internal complaints and infectious diseases'. From their analysis, they attempted to design an ideal multi-faceted sickroom which would meet the needs of the children of the different age groups, and, out of this, to organize care-groups, and finally wards. They remained convinced, however, that 'concerning the question of children's hospitals,' there 'will continue to be differing opinions'.

By this time, the old idea of the outpatient unit had been practically abandoned, even though Bessau had stressed as late as 1928 that 'outpatient clinics acting as university teaching hospitals' are 'an absolute must'. In institutions not affiliated with a university, the issue had become a problem of professional politics. Bessau was nevertheless of the opinion that one should continue to support the concept of an outpatient department, and to be able to say of the medical directors: 'Ye shall know them by their out-patient departments'.[26]

The opening of this paper posed the deceptively simple question: Why, to what end, and in what form were institutions for sick children established? Based on our historical analysis, we are now in a position to propose the following reply.

The reason for children's hospitals coming into being must be linked to the coincidence of the rise of Enlightenment values, leading to public protection of children on the one hand, and the interest of the medical profession in exploiting the children in the service of its new scientific orientation on the other.

Consequently, the end or purpose of the children's hospital was never strictly bound up only with the effort to advance clinical knowledge, to teach students, and to cure diseases, but had as much to do with society's growing interest in its children as social resources, to be entrusted to medical care for individual and social survival.

The development of the structure and the functioning of the children's hospital vacillated between the self-interest of the medical profession and the proper needs of the sick children. The history of this institution thus reflects both these competing factors at every time, if in very different forms.

Given all these competing forces shaping the history of the children's hospital, we are left with no 'ideal model' of the institution, neither in its outward appearance nor in its inner organization. Indeed, I am personally convinced that the search after such an 'ideal type' must be ultimately fruitless, because in the end the needs of a sick child are not met simply through institutionalized cure and care.

Notes

1. I am grateful to Dr Anne Harrington for her assistance in the English translation and revision of this paper.
2. E. Seidler, 'Das kranke Kind. Historische Modelle einer Medizinischen Anthropologie des Kindesalters', in J. Martin and A. Nitschke (eds), *Zur Sozialgeschichte der Kindheit. Historische Anthropologie*, vol. 4 (Freiburg/München, 1986), 685–709.
3. D. Jetter, *Grundzüge der Krankenhausgeschichte (1800–1900)* (Darmstadt, 1977).
4. G. Fr. Still, *The History of Pediatrics* (London, 1965), 422. See also W.J. Maloney, *George and John Armstrong of Castleton: Two Eighteenth-Century Medical Pioneers* (Edinburgh, 1954); F.N.L. Poynter, 'A unique copy of George Armstrong's printed proposals for establishing the dispensary for sick children, London 1769', *Medical History*, 1 (1957), 65–6.
5. G. Armstrong, 'A general account of the dispensary for the relief of the infant poor', in *An Account of the Diseases Most Incident to Children, from the Birth till the Age of Puberty, with a Successful Method of Treating Them*, new edn (London, 1783), 179–200.
6. Op. cit., p. 197.
7. Ch. West, *On Hospital Organisation, with Special Reference to the Organisation of Hospitals for Children* (London, 1877).
8. H. Dorschel, *Die frühe Wiener Pädiatrie* (Med. thesis, Heidelberg, 1957).
9. P. Vallery-Radot, *Deux siècles d'histoire hospitalière de Henri IV à Louis-Philippe (1802–1836)* (Paris, 1947).
10. J.R. Tenon, *Mémoires sur les hôpitaux de Paris* (Paris, 1788).
11. E.H. Ackerknecht, *Medicine in the Paris Hospital, 1794–1848* (Baltimore, 1966).
12. C.A. Wunderlich, *Wien und Paris. Ein Beitrag zur Geschichte und Beurtheilung der gegenwärtigen Heilkunde* (Stuttgart, 1841).
13. K. Rauchfuss, 'Die Kinderheilanstalten', in Carl Gerhardt (ed.), *Handbuch der Kinderkrankheiten*, vol. 1 (Tübingen, 1877), 463–528.
14. F.S. Hügel, *Beschreibung sämmtlicher Kinderheilanstalten in Europa. Nebst einer Anleitung zur zweckmässigen Organisation von Kinder-Krankeninstituten und Kinderspitälern, mit Beiträgen zur Geschichte und Reform sämmtlicher Spitäler im Allgemeinen* (Wien, 1848).
15. Rauchfuss, 'Kinderheilanstalten'.
16. ibid.
17. F. Nightingale, *Notes on Hospitals*, 3rd edn (London, 1863), p. 124.

18. See P. Wunderlich, 'Arthur Schlossmann (1867–1932) und die Kinderheilkunde in Dresden', in H. Schadewaldt (ed.), *Düsseldorfer Arbeiten zur Geschichte der Medizin*, vol. 27 (Düsseldorf, 1967), pp. ix–xxiv.

19. J.G. Rey, 'Anstalten und Einrichtungen für Kinder', in Philipp Biedert (ed.), *Das Kind, seine geistige und körperliche Pflege von der Geburt bis zur Reife* (Stuttgart, 1906), 176–88.

20. *Monatsschrift für Kinderheilkunde* (Beiträge der Jahresversammlung 1928 der Deutschen Gesellschaft für Kinderheilkunde in Hamburg) 41 (1928), 227–306.

21. E. Feer, 'Bau und Einrichtung der Kinderkrankenhauses', in op. cit., 227–41.

22. A. Schlossmann, 'Uber die Versorgun infektionskranker Kinder', in op. cit., 261–300.

23. *Das Krankenhaus. Zeitschrift für das gesamte Krankenhauswesen.* Sonderheft: *Das Kind im Krankenhaus*, 49 (1957), Heft 9, 366-436.

24. G. Fanconi, 'Der Bau von Kinderkrankenhäusern ausserhalb Deutschlands', in op. cit., 370–1.

25. J. Wolff and H. Sahl, 'Das Kinderkrankenhaus', op. cit., 372–416.

26. G. Bessau, 'Das Ambulanzproblem', in *Monatsschrift für Kinderheilkunde*, 301–6.

8

'Fame and fortune by means of bricks and mortar': the medical profession and specialist hospitals in Britain, 1800–1948

Lindsay Granshaw

Early nineteenth-century medical specialists in Britain were often regarded by others in their profession as little more than quacks. They guarded their secret potions jealously, it was said, and sought to make large amounts of money out of the gullible. Yet by the time of the First World War specialists were among the leaders in the profession, associating with royals, and vying with each other in the possession of expensive cars. (Albeit some cynics remarked that they kept their remedies to themselves, and made large amounts of money out of the gullible.)[1]

How did the specialist establish himself on the pinnacle of the profession? Or was he already there, at least in the eyes of the public, if not in those of fellow doctors? Certainly there were a number of well-established specialists in the early nineteenth century with upper-class patrons.[2] But the power and position of specialists as a group was largely a later thing – and in Britain the special hospitals played a key role in that transition. Many of these mostly nineteenth-century creations enabled medical men, in the *British Medical Journal*'s words, to 'step to fame and fortune by means of bricks and mortar'.[3] That they were such a route to power, prestige, and wealth is underlined by the vociferous opposition they encountered from much of the medical profession in the mid-nineteenth century.

Certainly the developments in the theory and practice of medicine emanating from Paris in the early nineteenth century, shifting focus from the body as an indivisible whole to a composite of parts, emphasizing particular organs as the seats of disease, did nothing to hinder the growth of – often specialized – hospitals.[4] However, founders of the hospitals rarely made reference to such changing ideas, and the hospitals usually preceded the development of specialist fields. In most cases, too, they preceded the development of specialized instruments; the invention of particular tools cannot be seen as the reason for the massive expansion in the number and range of special hospitals.[5] It was in the assistance that the hospitals provided to the upwardly-mobile doctor that the key to their foundation can be found.

Special hospitals played a larger part than simply allowing their founders to establish their own reputations. They enabled those on the edge of the profession to gain a crucial place within it. They helped to crystallize the divisions between hospital doctors and general practitioners. They provided a central focus for the profession's struggle to oust lay control from hospitals.[6] In most instances, too, special hospitals were medicalized earlier than general hospitals – medical men spent longer there, patients underwent more medical intervention (especially surgical), and regulations were geared far more to medical work.[7] Condemned by most of the profession when first established, by the end of the century those who might realistically aspire to be leaders in the profession applied to join the staffs of the special hospitals. It was from the special hospitals, too, that textbooks, articles, and novel procedures appeared, defining new fields and emphasizing – always – the necessity of taking specialist advice.

But first it is important to stress that whatever medical men may have thought of so-called quacks in the eighteenth century, the public did not necessarily agree. As Roy Porter has argued, the regulars might talk of how quacks undermined the profession, but that did not stop them prospering; the public seemed quite happy to use their services, or to spread their custom between various practitioners, regular or otherwise.[8] The specialists in the early nineteenth century were very anxious, however, to reject the label of quackery, and they in their turn condemned those whom they considered to be quacks.[9] None of this professional rivalry necessarily had a major impact on potential patients. Quacks prospered – or not – along with the rest.

Thus, specialization had long been the means by which outsiders in medicine might seek to rise. However, it took a much more institutionalized form in the nineteenth century, as institutions themselves became more important to the nascent medical profession. Hospitals in the nineteenth century became the profession's training ground, the main area in which lay control was rejected, the workplace of the medical elite, and, later, the places in which 'scientific medicine', so important to the image of the profession, could in theory be practised.[10] Given the increasing importance of hospitals to the British medical profession, it is not surprising that the new specialists took the hospital route in their attempts to establish themselves.

The middle and upper classes were treated at home in the eighteenth and nineteenth century; hospitals were supposed to be only for the 'deserving poor'. They were supported through philanthropy, and lay men and women received social kudos along with such governors' rights as patient admission and staff selection. This powerful lay influence far from deterred medical men from hospital involvement: rather it encouraged them. They were anxious to secure hospital positions, with the important contacts with the rich and powerful that these brought.[11]

By the end of the eighteenth century there were a number of hospitals in Britain, mostly in the major towns. Set up by laymen, they reflected the growth of the bourgeoisie with its interest in philanthropy. Such hospitals usually excluded certain types of patients, such as lunatics, incurables, and women in childbirth, but at mid-century a few hospitals such as lying-in charities were set up for some of these excluded groups.[12] Again, they were largely lay foundations.

From the last third of the eighteenth century there was a new development – the foundation of medical institutions, mostly outpatient dispensaries, by medical men. The first, the Aldersgate Street Dispensary, established by John Lettsom in 1770, set a trend. Lettsom, a Quaker, was disaffected with the medical establishment that dominated London medicine, and his two foundations, the dispensary and the Medical Society of London, were expressions of that dissatisfaction.[13] A number of dispensaries were set up, particularly in the cities, at the end of the eighteenth century and into the nineteenth century, mostly by medical men.[14]

The specialist hospitals of the nineteenth century usually began as outpatient dispensaries and were an outgrowth of this development. The pattern of their establishment and their use by both the medical men and patients differed significantly from that of the general hospitals. It was crucially important that they were set up not by lay philanthropists but by medical men. Almost invariably these medical men were ambitious entrepreneurs, but something of outsiders, unable to secure the central positions that they desired within the medical profession. Professionalization was one method of assuring position in a rapidly changing world, a route taken by the doctors. As they sought to control entry to their group and to monitor behaviour within it, they also reinforced their tenet that it was inappropriate to advertise. Ways around that had always been found, and a hospital position served as just such a good advertisement, since patients knew that a hospital doctor had at least the right connections.[15] Hospital positions, though, were available only to a few. For doctors to secure hospital positions in the early nineteenth century, it was necessary either to gain medical patronage or to 'buy' the governors who voted in hospital elections, and that could be a very expensive business. At the Aldersgate Street Dispensary in 1824, for example, two competing applicants paid 600 guineas between them in the hope of being elected as surgeon – and of course one failed and had to try again. These were men who were just starting out in practice.[16]

The medical routes to public notice were largely monopolized by those who were already moving in the right social circles. There were other ways – the brass plates, notices giving a change of address, joining the masons (an increasingly useful route to prosperity it seemed), joining local societies and clubs.[17] Unable to advertise directly, it was those who were outside the inner circles but whose intention was to gain admission who took the route of specialization. Upwardly mobile entrepreneurs were as evident in the medical profession as in other social strands of nineteenth-century life. The foundation of special hospitals became a way for some of these medical men to break through.

The template for nineteenth-century special hospitals was Moorfields, set up by John Cunningham Saunders in 1804 as the London Dispensary for the Relief of the Poor Afflicted with Ear and Eye Diseases.[18] Saunders was able and ambitious but his family did not come from sufficiently influential circles. However, he was by no means a complete outsider and had established a foothold on the bottom of the hospital ladder. What was critical was that he could not then climb all the way up it. Saunders was born not in London but in Devon, in 1773. He was apprenticed locally to a barber surgeon. Having served his five years, he came to London to walk the wards so that he could practise in the metropolis, the aim of many an ambitious provincial surgeon. He became house-pupil to Astley Cooper, then a lecturer at St Thomas's, no doubt paying for the privilege.[19] Through Cooper's patronage he secured the position of demonstrator of anatomy at St Thomas's. He also acted as Cooper's dresser. So far, Saunders was doing very well. However, in 1800 Astley Cooper was appointed on his uncle's retirement as surgeon at Guy's, the hospital which both partnered and rivalled St Thomas's.[20] Cooper took on Benjamin Travers as his apprentice, a favoured position from which the patron often arranged promotion. In due course Travers became a surgeon at St Thomas's.[21] (In later years Astley Cooper similarly favoured a range of former apprentices as well as relatives.[22]) John Cunningham Saunders can therefore have had little realistic prospect of Cooper's patronage for the more important positions, and in 1801 he left London for the provinces. However, he soon decided to return to his earlier ambition of securing a practice in the capital, and resumed his position as demonstrator of anatomy at St Thomas's.[23] Saunders was to move no further up the hierarchy.

Astley Cooper had a particular interest in the anatomy of the ear, and Saunders exploited his connection with him by emphasizing a degree of specialization in diseases of the ear, on which he published a book.[24] Saunders then went a stage further in this professional manner of self-advertisement: he established his dispensary for treating ear and eye diseases. Within a few months it was concentrating on eye diseases alone, and Saunders had converted his dispensary into an infirmary with a few beds. He now began to compile a book on diseases of the eye, based upon the cases he saw at his hospital.[25] This is a pattern also seen in later establishments; the medical men wrote what they emphasized were 'practical treatises' (which were accessible both to an educated public and to other doctors) which served to stress their specialist skills, and to differentiate them from the quacks with their secret remedies. However, before Saunders' book could be published, he died, at the age of 37, in 1810.[26]

The early success of John Cunningham Saunders' enterprise acted as immediate encouragement to other establishments. A colleague of Saunders enlisted the help of a banker in setting up an eye hospital in Exeter in 1808, this was followed by Dr. Goldwyer setting up a hospital in Bristol (1810), Dr Sims in Bath (1811), Mr. W.J. Wilson, an oculist, in Manchester (1814), a surgeon, Ryall, setting up an eye and ear hospital in Dublin (1814), and Dr Guthrie establishing a second London eye hospital (1816). Thus, all were set up by medical men. In the subsequent two decades, eye hospitals were established in Shrewsbury, Liverpool, Plymouth, Newcastle, Norwich, Birmingham, Glasgow, Brighton, Edinburgh, Aberdeen, Weymouth, and Sunderland.[27]

Besides the eye hospitals, there were a handful of other infirmaries which specialized in the treatment of other parts of the body. For example, in 1814 Dr Isaac Buxton set up in London what became the Royal Hospital for Diseases of the Chest, and an orthopaedic hospital was set up in Birmingham in 1817. However, the few other specialist institutions established between 1815 and 1835 were far outnumbered by the highly successful formula, the eye hospital.[28] From the 1830s that began to change. One of the next group of hospitals, diversifying away from eye hospitals and again acting as an exemplar for later establishments, was the Fistula Infirmary, which became St Mark's Hospital in London.[29]

As in the case of Moorfields, the Fistula Infirmary was founded by a surgeon from the provinces, in this case Bath. Frederick Salmon had been apprenticed to a local surgeon-apothecary, then came to London in 1817 to complete his training at St Bartholomew's, where he walked the wards, with ninety-two other pupils, behind John Abernethy.[30] Salmon then paid him more than 8 guineas to become his house surgeon, before trying to set up a practice in London. Failing to get on the staff of the Aldersgate Street Dispensary, in 1825 he learned that Abernethy was intending to retire from Bart's and endeavoured to secure his support to be his replacement. It then emerged that Abernethy had made an arrangement with another former pupil for him to take his position, on the written understanding that he in turn passed the position on to Abernethy's young son. In the ensuing controversy, fuelled by the newly-established *Lancet*, Abernethy certainly came under criticism, but Salmon did not gain thereby – he did not secure appointment.[31] Salmon finally succeeded in being appointed at the Aldersgate Street Dispensary in 1827, only to lose the position again in 1833 when all the staff resigned in protest at the controlling hand of the lay governors.[32]

Frederick Salmon had already begun to specialize – in the treatment of rectal diseases – and had published two books on the subject.[33] (Significantly he published nothing further after he had established his hospital; his fame as a rectal specialist was now such that he did not need to do so, and he left that to others on the staff of his hospital in later years.) Salmon had joined a businessmen's club in the City of London, where he had established his practice, and it was from there that he recruited his philanthropic helpers. The founders of specialist hospitals discovered, to the irritation of others in the profession, that there was no shortage of lay philanthropic help in getting their institutions going – if they showed the right entrepreneurial skills.[34] The equally upwardly mobile middle-class traders, lawyers, and business-men regarded public philanthropy as confirming or convey-ing on them recognition of their position in the social scale.

Salmon established his institution as a tiny dispensary in one room in the City of London. His enterprise flourished and in the 1850s a thirty-bedded hospital was built. By the time of Salmon's death in 1868 there were four surgeons on the staff. Founded as the Benevolent Dispensary for the Relief of the Poor Afflicted with Fistula, Piles, and other Diseases of the Rectum and Lower Intestines, it had by the early 1850s become St Mark's Hospital.[35] (It had become commonplace for the special hospitals to take saints' names – any saint's name – as they sought greater respectability.[36])

The 1830s saw, besides the Fistula Infirmary, the establish-ment by local doctors of an Eye, Ear, and Throat Infirmary in Edinburgh, and the Hospital for the Cure of Deformities by Drs W.J. Little and Quarles Harris (later the Royal, then the Royal National, Orthopaedic Hospital), and the Metropolitan Institution for Diseases of the Ear, Throat, and Vocal Organs, founded by Drs Ordwin, Walsh, Everett,

Streeton, and Stephenson. In the 1840s and 1850s the trend became even more marked, with the foundation in London of two hospitals for consumption including the Brompton Hospital, the Women's Hospital in Soho, the Cancer Hospital, the Hospital for Sick Children, Great Ormond Street, and several hospitals for skin diseases, diseases of the chest, and orthopaedic problems.[37] Outside London more eye hospitals were set up, as well as hospitals for women and children, ear and throat complaints, consumption, and a dental hospital. By the early 1860s there were at least sixty-six special institutions in London alone.[38]

Special hospitals were relatively easy to establish: the practitioner usually rented a house or just a couple of rooms, and installed a few beds in the care of a residential 'matron' and perhaps a house surgeon. The success or failure of the institution then usually turned on whether the founder could attract and then retain sufficient charitable interest. Many little institutions went under within a few years of being set up, or else their founders secured other appointments and let their enterprises fold. Attracting patients never seemed to be a problem, and this patient demand underlay the overall success of the specialist hospital movement.[39]

Patients might be happy, but the medical profession was not. They held very mixed feelings about the specialists and their hospitals, with the disruption of the *status quo* that this implied. Those at the top of the medical hierarchy resented their positions being undermined. As teaching became increasingly important at the general hospitals, it was argued that the proliferation of special hospitals drew away interesting cases from the schools. General practitioners had even greater reason to fear the special hospitals. They argued that it was not just the very poor who were turning to the multiplying hospitals but those who were slightly better-off – in other words, their own patients.

Defending both hospital doctor and general practitioner, the *British Medical Journal* made its attitude very clear in a campaign it ran against special hospitals in the early 1860s. As it put it:

> it would appear that [these] hospitals . . . were effected
> solely on the behalf of suffering humanity . . . . Anyone
> who knows anything of the working of our metropolitan

charitable institutions is fully aware how far this is from
the real – and we must add . . . the vulgar – truth.[40]

Most of the specialist hospitals were established through 'the
energetic action of some individual'.[41] They would begin as
a dispensary; an energetic surgeon then 'makes up his mind
to step to fame and fortune by means of bricks and
mortar'.[42] First he must decide on some 'striking specialty'
such as the treatment of 'inverted eyelashes'. A quiet house
was taken in a side street,

> patrons and patronesses are canvassed for, and in an
> incredibly short space of time a goodly sprinkling of the
> aristocracy have been found to pledge themselves to
> serve suffering humanity and Mr. —, in the matter of
> inverted eyelashes.[43]

'Carefully got up statistics' would then prove that every tenth
person was suffering from this terrible disease, with 20,000
cases treated a year, and the dispensary would need to be
expanded into a hospital. Although inverted eyelashes could
be treated 'in the old established hospital close at hand', this
would never be realized by the gentlemen and ladies

> who so obsequiously follow the lead of the ambitious Mr.
> —, who is determined that there shall be a building
> devoted to nothing but misplaced eyelashes and perhaps
> – but this is of course quite under the rose – to
> himself.[44]

To the *British Medical Journal*, special hospitals served no
useful purpose at all. They starved the general hospitals of
the kind of cases which were so instructive to medical
students, they destroyed 'that unity of disease which the
philosophic mind should always keep in mind'; and they
squandered public funds.[45] Special hospitals 'will never
furnish great surgeons, or advance the art beyond mere
manipulative smartness'.[46]

No sooner had the *British Medical Journal* issued this
complaint than it heard that a 'hospital for stone' was about
to be established.[47] The British Medical Association (BMA)
initiated – with some dissension – a petition against all

special hospitals. One dissenter had himself condemned special hospitals six years earlier, but he had subsequently joined one; he now maintained that he would 'give up his post tomorrow if he saw an indication of liberal reform in the greater institutions'.[48] In other words, if he could gain an appointment at a major hospital, his allegiance to special hospitals would immediately evaporate. From his new position he now held that opposition stoked up by the *British Medical Journal* was selfish, exclusive, and hypocritical. However, a more typical view was put by another practitioner who argued that special hospitals were established for one purpose only – the self-interest of their founder. 'It was true that the gentlemen engaged in these hospitals got their names spread all over England, but in the meantime the profession was being ruined.'[49] He complained that they drew patients from all over the country, yet made no investigation whatsoever of whether they were indeed worthy recipients of charity; in other words, whether they were too poor to have afforded to pay a local doctor. The only permissible special institutions, it was maintained, were those which treated cases which were not admitted to general hospitals. An example quoted was epilepsy: Brown-Séquard had moved from Paris to become a surgeon at the National Hospital for the Paralysed and Epileptic, Queen Square; as a rationalization or not, he argued that 'when cases of epilepsy were received into general hospitals, he would resign his situation at once'.[50]

Opposing the new hospital for stone, a manifesto was signed by many of the senior physicians and surgeons on the staffs of general hospitals, stating that they were of the opinion

> that much detriment to the public and the medical profession arises from the modern practice of opening small institutions, under the name of hospitals, for particular forms of disease, in the treatment of which no other management, appliance or attention is required than is already supplied in the existing general hospitals.[51]

They emphasized that a hospital for the treatment of stone and diseases of the urinary organs was 'especially unnecessary'.[52]

The subject continued to be much debated, with a few protagonists arguing that medical knowledge had advanced to a stage where specialization was necessary, others that special institutions were far more expensive in their care for patients than the general hospitals. The hospital for stone went ahead and in 1864 was named St Peter's Hospital. The *British Medical Journal* wondered whether the particular saint had been selected as a joke. The hospital was also dedicated to the treatment of urinary diseases. 'Urinary diseases!' exclaimed the journal: 'all the medical world knows what *they* mean in the eyes of the enlightened public'.[53] Indeed the surgeons at St Peter's in the later nineteenth century had flourishing venereal disease practices among the aristocracy – one, Sir Alfred Cooper, father-in-law of Lady Diana Cooper, travelled round London in what was known as his 'clap trap'.[54]

St Peter's Hospital was set up at a turning point for special hospitals. There was considerable pressure on their founders and their members of staff to abandon their enterprises – pressure which came from both hospital doctors and general practitioners. The general hospitals were just beginning to try to undermine the specialist institutions by appointing specialists themselves, at least in the treatment of eye diseases, and setting aside beds for special cases. However the development of specialist hospitals seemed unstoppable. Many hospital doctors themselves already had profitable associations with them. Most crucially, public support, both from patients and philanthropists, was considerable, even if the controversies of the 1860s show clearly the pulls in the different directions.

St Peter's illustrates the case well. St Peter's had two founder surgeons, Armstrong Todd and Thomas Spencer Wells. Todd seems to have been the mover behind the project. He was Irish and had graduated from Dublin. He became surgeon to the Marylebone Dispensary, but he held no higher position – he was typical of other hospital founders. Wells was not. He was far better known. He was already actively involved in another special hospital, the Samaritan Hospital for Women. However, his operation of ovariotomy was far from accepted, and he stood somewhat outside the medical elite at the time. His public profile, though, was high and he served as a useful publicist for the new hospital. It was Wells who was given the task of drawing up the circular which set forth the advantages of the new specialist hospital.

At this stage, he clearly felt that it was appropriate to be involved in such an enterprise. Within two years, though, he had resigned; St Peter's had become the focus of too much professional discontent.[55]

A second case at St Peter's shows the outcome eventually going the other way. In 1864 Walter Coulson, then surgical registrar at St Mary's Hospital, became surgeon at St Peter's. Coulson's uncle was a prominent and successful medical practitioner, with an interest in urinary diseases. Armstrong Todd at St Peter's, having lost Spencer Wells, encouraged Coulson to join him. The surgical staff at St Mary's immediately condemned St Peter's as 'useless and mischievous, an injury to the schools and an insult to the hospitals'.[56] Coulson saw where his greater interest lay at that stage and resigned his position at St Peter's; he was duly rewarded in 1866 by being appointed assistant surgeon at St Mary's. However, he then resumed his position at St Peter's, and his colleagues at St Mary's were up in arms. They wrote to the medical press in protest. Coulson responded by pointing out that two of the St Mary's surgeons were on the staff of the Lock Hospital and that one of these, James R. Lane, was on the staff of St Mark's as well.[57] Reflecting the gravity of the row, Lane promptly resigned from St. Mark's. The *British Medical Journal* recorded that Lane had 'withdrawn' from the office of surgeon at St Mark's, adding that 'The institution is one which finds small favour in the eyes of the profession now.'[58] Reflecting reality, though, the journal remarked that there would be applicants for the vacancy, 'unenviable as the post may now be generally considered'[59] – such was the demand for such positions, whatever the medical establishment might say.

Coulson did not see special hospitals in the same light as the *BMJ*, however. He refused to be dislodged from St Peter's, remaining there until his death in 1889. St Peter's became embroiled in similar controversies: a Middlesex surgeon, Thomas Nunn, was elected to the staff in the same traumatic year, 1866, but resigned barely a year later because of pressure from the Middlesex. In doing so he recorded that he resigned 'in order to prevent being forced into open rupture with several of my colleagues at the Middlesex Hospital with whom I have been connected nearly twenty years'.[60]

The poor view of special hospitals among the establishment was expressed by the medical press in the obituaries of Frederick Salmon in 1868. The *Lancet* was somewhat more favourable than the *British Medical Journal*, reflecting a gradually differing readership; it recorded the establishment of St Mark's thus: 'The step met with great professional opposition; but by indomitable perseverance, obtaining large funds from the public for the support of the institution, he ultimately succeeded'.[61] Specialization had clearly resulted in great material benefits to Salmon, and the *Lancet* noted that he 'had a large share of private practice in the diseases which he made his especial study'.[62] The *British Medical Journal* hardly beat about the bush:

How far the course which he took was prompted by difficulties in pursuing a useful and honourable career in a general hospital, where his labours would have been more useful and more instructive, it is now difficult to say. It was, we fully believe, contrary to the best interests both of the profession and of the public; and the success of St Mark's Hospital was of unfortunate omen, and has since borne fruit in encouraging similar enterprises.[63]

For the *British Medical Journal* and those whom the journal sought to represent, however, it was already a lost cause. The pressures supporting specialist hospitals were proving far stronger than those restraining them. The staff who joined well-established, wealthily-patronized hospitals were now rarely outsiders. Some resigned their special hospital positions after a few years, when they were well-established in private practice, while retaining their general hospital positions. Occasionally, though infrequently, they gave up their general hospital position and retained only their specialist affiliation. The variety of patterns can be seen at St Mark's. Peter Gowlland, for example, reacted very differently from his immediate contemporary, James Lane; where Lane, under pressure from St Mary's, gave up the position at St Mark's, Gowlland on the other hand relinquished his London Hospital position to concentrate only on rectal diseases – and died a rich man as a result.[64] A few prominent men did not seek a teaching hospital position even though they would have stood an excellent chance of obtaining one. The leading surgeon at St Mark's with the largest practice in rectal diseases in London, William Allingham, author of the main textbook on the subject, winner of numerous prizes during his training at St Thomas's, member of the Council of the Royal College of Surgeons, never held a position at a teaching hospital.[65]

Mixed feelings about specialist hospitals continued to be voiced in the last third of the nineteenth century. When the House of Lords in the 1890s conducted an enquiry into the state of the metropolitan hospitals, many of the medical men giving evidence argued against specialist institutions: such hospitals drained resources from more worthy recipients, let alone stealing their patients.[66] However, despite such rhetoric, there is much evidence that the professional elite were now exploiting the special hospitals. A new pattern in the use of the specialist hospitals by the doctors was emerging. While some of the surgeons and physicians emphasized one specialty only, by the turn of the century those climbing the ladder turned from one specialty to another, in rapid succession. In many cases, biographies and histories indicate that they made no contribution to any specialty. However, they did develop thriving private practices and frequently gained appointments at the teaching hospitals after they had gained experience at the specialist institutions.

Taking a sample of 500 medical men between 1850 and 1950 who were Fellows of the Royal College of Surgeons, therefore recorded in Plarr and likely to be among the elite, the changing pattern in associations with special hospitals can be seen. Plarr under-estimates, since there are a number within the sample where the 'life' does not mention a link with a special hospital which other sources reveal. After all, even if a medical man regarded it as important to his initial career to join such a hospital, at a later date he might obscure this, or others would find it insignificant, and obituaries would fail to record an early association. However, within that constraint, instructive information emerges. In the 1850s about 20 per cent of those in Plarr are recorded to have had some association with a special hospital. Often this was a temporary link, although some founders of hospitals are numbered amongst them. Between the 1860s and the 1880s the proportion rose to 25 per cent, but from the 1890s right through and into the National Health Service it rose to just under 60 per cent.[67]

Thus it was not just the outsiders in the profession who were using the special hospitals, but many of those who could reasonably expect bright futures. Certainly some with humble origins still found the specialist hospital route profitable, but others hardly needed such a boost, and yet sought such positions. Examples illustrating these points can be given. Someone who started on an outside track, Sir John Bland-Sutton, but who became a much famed early twentieth-century cancer surgeon at the Middlesex Hospital, came from a large family in which 'money was not too abundant' and had to teach to keep himself afloat.[68] He did not have powerful connections, and

> he climbed the ladder by ordinary steps, slowly at first as a junior demonstrator of anatomy, then as curator of the hospital museum, next as assistant surgeon to a small special hospital, finally as assistant surgeon, surgeon and consulting surgeon to his own hospital, the Middlesex.[69]

The assumption was that his special hospital appointment was part of his rise to fame and fortune.

Sir Henry Butlin, surgeon at St Bartholomew's and subsequently President of the Royal College of Surgeons, again from inauspicious origins, had traced a similar path.[70] Percy Furnivall, Sir Henry's son-in-law, and well-connected, in the 1890s acted as clinical assistant to a children's hospital, an eye hospital, and a throat hospital, joined the staff of the Metropolitan Hospital, then St Mark's, until finally securing a position at the London Hospital, after which he dropped his remaining specialist positions. He hardly needed a boost to his position, and yet he saw the special hospital affiliation as dispensable but important.[71]

Perhaps most revealing is the Bickersteth family, of Liverpool, who became prominent in the medical profession in the nineteenth century. An eighteenth-century Bickersteth had come from a distinguished social background, and had had a large medical practice in Kirkby Lonsdale, Westmorland. His son, Robert (1787–1857), trained in the best school of the time, Edinburgh, then went to London, before returning north to become surgeon to the Liverpool Infirmary in 1810, which he used as a base for building up a very successful practice.[72] Robert Bickersteth's son, Edward (1828–1908), followed him through Edinburgh, went on to St Bartholomew's, then made a medical tour of Dublin and did what all bright, wealthy young doctors hoped to do, spent some time in Paris before returning to Liverpool where he succeeded his father as surgeon to the Infirmary in 1857.[73] Edward Bickersteth's son, Robert Alexander (1862–1924), took the route that had become the most select in the closing decades of the nineteenth century. He was sent to Eton, Cambridge, and then St Bartholomew's, where he qualified in the early 1890s. With everything in his favour, he chose as his next step to act as clinical assistant first at the Throat Hospital, Golden Square, and then at Moorfields. Only after this did he return to Liverpool, where he took up the position of surgeon to the Royal Liverpool Infirmary. Here his interest was in yet a third specialty, urology. It had clearly been seen both by Bickersteth and his advisers that part of his training should be gained at the special hospitals.[74]

The surgeons who joined the specialist institutions at the end of the nineteenth century fell into two main categories: those who regarded them as stepping stones to large private practices or general hospital appointments; and those who were the more dedicated specialists. It was the latter group that now pushed their chosen fields outwards, publishing first for general practitioners, warning them of the dangers of non-specialist treatment, and then by the early twentieth century for colleagues in their own fields. Journals, clubs, and societies began to be set up in the different fields. It was these specialists, too, who developed new operations, differentiated between diseases, and devised novel instruments.[75]

This evolving pattern did not stop members of the medical profession retaining their very mixed feelings about the idea of specializing at all. As if in pursuit of the image of the classically-educated nineteenth-century doctor with the Renaissance mind, many of the most socially prominent medical men continued to strive for success in general surgery or general medicine, whatever the financial rewards of specialization.[76] The First World War acted as a further stimulus to specialization and to the importance of the special hospitals to medical men. Many doctors went to France, finding on their return that former patients and medical contacts were lost. Specialization was one way of re-establishing a reasonable practice.[77] But the generalist ideal persisted; as one returning surgeon, Sir Charles Gordon-Watson, ruefully saw it, even though he was on the staff of St Bartholomew's, it was his link with a special hospital which was now important:

> How thankful I am that I practised general surgery for many years before the inevitable current of specialisation washed me into this back water. There save for an occasional excursion into the main stream, I must needs stay 'put' to the end, though not unthankful for the rewards that it brings and the benefits that I have been able to hand out to many sufferers.[78]

Clearly, if he had been able to, he would have stayed a general surgeon.

It was the National Health Service, set up in 1948, though, that took at face value the criticisms of the special hospitals. Organized around district general and general teaching hospitals, with specialist departments, many of the specialist hospitals were swallowed up.[79] As ever, the medical profession seemed to agree that specialist institutions were not wanted. As the *Lancet* put it in 1961:

> the small special hospital, which was so perfect an instrument sixty years ago, when individuals were developing their subjects on their own, is no longer the ideal place in an era in which teamwork and the laboratory have taken the place of the single-handed clinician or surgeon.[80]

Ironically, there seemed to have been no period, despite the *Lancet*'s assumption, when special hospitals were agreed to be useful institutions. And yet special hospitals had served the interests of those excluded from elite positions, whose abilities as entrepreneurs rivalled any others in Victorian society. As social changes disrupted the *status quo*, they fought for advancement through establishing their own institutions, adopting the forms of regular medicine. The battles against such specialization were intense, but general practitioners were in a weak position to resist, and although hospital surgeons and physicians for many years opposed special hospitals, the younger generations who formed the future elite found them useful. Their success – based on popular support – was by and large so great that it only took a generation or so before those who could expect to be the elite in the profession were laying aside former disapproval and seeking to join the specialist institutions. Many remained remarkably ambivalent about specialization, so that in the 1870s and 1880s specialist positions were usually relinquished once a surgeon or physician was well established. By the end of the century that was less likely to be the case – an increasing number of those on the staffs of the specialist hospitals now stayed with that specialty throughout their working lives, originating in their fields so that in turn they attracted new entrants into these areas. But for many others, though specialization seemed part of their career pattern, they retained the earlier disdain for such 'narrow-mindedness'. They joined the staff, hoping to enhance their reputations and develop a clientele of patients in a particular field, at least as a starting point, but a main aim of many was to be considered a generalist. Praised or berated, by the end of the nineteenth century and certainly in the twentieth century, therefore, special hospitals were – like the general hospitals earlier in the century – serving the interests of the elite.

Notes

1. For the flourishing twentieth-century specialists, see R. Pound, *Harley Street* (Michael Joseph, London, 1967).

2. R. Porter, 'Before the fringe', in R. Cooter (ed.), *Alternatives; The Social History of Alternative Medicine* (Macmillan, London, 1988).

3. 'Hospital distress', *British Medical Journal*, no. 1 (1860), 458.

4. For varying accounts of the impact of Paris medicine, see M. Foucault, *The Birth of the Clinic. An Archaeology of Medical Perception*, trans. A.M. Sheridan (Tavistock, London, 1976); E. Ackerknecht, *Medicine at the Paris Hospital, 1794–1848* (The Johns Hopkins Press, Baltimore, 1967); and T. Gelfand, *Professionalizing Modern Medicine; Paris Surgeons and Medical Science and Institutions in the 18th Century* (Greenwood Press, Westport, Connecticut, 1980).

5. G. Rosen, *Specialization of Medicine* (Froben Press, New York, 1944) particularly emphasized that instruments played a major role in the development of specialized medicine.

6. See M. Jeanne Peterson, *The Medical Profession in Mid-Victorian London* (University of California Press, Berkeley, 1978) for the

battles against lay control. For professionalization, see E. Freidson, *Profession of Medicine* (Dodd, Mead, New York, 1970); E. Freidson, *Professional Powers. A Study of the Institutionalisation of Formal Knowledge* (University of Chicago Press, Chicago and London, 1986); I. Waddington, *The Medical Profession in the Industrial Revolution* (Gill & Macmillan, Dublin, 1984); N. Parry and J. Parry, *The Rise of the Medical Profession* (Croom Helm, London, 1976). For the division between GP and hospital doctor, see F. Honigsbaum, *The Division in British Medicine: A History of the Separation of General Practice From Hospital Care, 1911–1968* (Kogan Page, London, 1979).

7. L. Granshaw, *St Mark's Hospital, London: A Social History of a Specialist Hospital* (King's Fund Historical Series, London, 1985).

8. R. Porter, 'Before the fringe'.

9. See for example F. Salmon, *Oration on the Necessity for an Entire Change in the Constitution and Government of the Royal College of Surgeons* (Whittaker, Treacher & Arnot, London, 1833). Salmon argues that the College should defend people like himself, though a specialist, and roundly condemned the quacks.

10. For the rhetoric or reality of scientific medicine, see C. Lawrence, 'Incommunicable knowledge: science, technology and the clinical art in Britain, 1850–1914', *Journal of Contemporary History*, no. 20 (1985), 503–20.

11. See, for example, the amounts of money involved in hospital elections in Granshaw, *St Mark's Hospital*, 11.

12. Brian Abel-Smith, *The Hospitals 1880-1948. A Study in Social Administration in England and Wales* (Heinemann, London, 1964); A. Gunn, 'Maternity hospitals', in F.N.L. Poynter (ed.), *The Evolution of Hospitals in Britain* (Pitman, London, 1964), 77–101; J. Woodward, *To Do The Sick No Harm. A Study of the British Voluntary Hospital System to 1875* (London, Routledge & Kegan Paul, 1974).

13. T. Hunt (ed.), *The Medical Society of London 1773–1973* (Heinemann, London, 1972).

14. Z. Cope, 'The history of the dispensary movement', in F.N.L. Poynter (ed.), *The Evolution of Hospitals in Britain* (Pitman, London, 1964).

15. Peterson, *The Medical Profession*.

16. See for example, 'The Westminster Medical Society and the resignation of the medical officers of the Aldersgate Street Dispensary', *Lancet*, no. 1 (1833–4), 218; 'General Dispensary Aldersgate Street', *Times*, 28 October 1833, 3; Veritas, 'Letter to the Editor', *Lancet*, no. 1 (1833–4), 340.

17. Peterson, *The Medical Profession*.

18. 'John Cunningham Saunders (1773–1810)', S. Lee (ed.) *Dictionary of National Biography*, vol. 17 (Smith, Elder, & Co., London, 1909), 815–16.

19. ibid.; B.B. Cooper, *The Life of Sir Astley Cooper*, 2 vols (John W. Parker, London, 1843); R.C. Brock, *The Life and Work of Astley Cooper* (E. & S. Livingstone, Edinburgh and London, 1952).

20. H.C. Cameron, *Mr Guy's Hospital, 1726–1948* (Longmans, Green & Co., London, 1954), 136–8.

21. F.G. Parsons, *The History of St Thomas's Hospital*, vol. 3 (Methuen, London, 1936), 243; E.M. McInnes, *St Thomas' Hospital* (George Allen & Unwin, London, 1963).

22. Peterson, *The Medical Profession*, 146–7, on Cooper's nephews.

23. *A Treatise on Some Practical Points relating to the Diseases of the Eye, by the late John Cunningham Saunders, Demonstrator of Anatomy at Saint Thomas's Hospital, Founder and Surgeon of the London Infirmary for Curing Diseases of the Eye to which are added, A Short Account of the Author's Life, and his Method of Curing the Congenital Cataract by his friend and colleague, J.R. Farre, M.D.* (Longman, Hurst, Rees, Orme & Brown, London 1816), 6–8; E. Treacher Collins, *The History and Tradition of the Moorfields Eye Hospital: One Hundred Years of Ophthalmic Discovery and Development* (H.K. Lewis & Co., London, 1929).

24. Saunders, *A Treatise*.

25. Farre, *A Short Account*, 14–15.

26. 'John Cunningham Saunders', *Dictionary of National Biography*; Farre, *A Short Account*, 13–35.

27. R. Kershaw, *Special Hospitals* (George Putnam & Sons, London, 1909), 62–4.

28. ibid.

29. Granshaw, *St Mark's Hospital*, 1–48.

30. Sir L. Harvey, *Journal*, 279, St Bartholomew's Hospital Archives, G/54.

31. 'Vacancy at St Bartholomew's', *Lancet*, vol. 12 (1826–7), 399–400; F. Salmon, 'Letter to the Editor,' *Lancet*, vol. 12 (1826–7), 474-5.

32. Granshaw, *St Mark's Hospital*, 13–14.

33. F. Salmon, *A Practical Essay on Stricture of the Rectum* (pr. James Bullock, London, 1828); Salmon, *Practical Observations on Prolapsus of the Rectum* (Whittaker, Treacher & Arnot, London, 1831).

34. Granshaw, *St Mark's Hospital*, 16–21.

35. Op. cit., p. 39.

36. See, for example, All Saints' Hospital, established by an Irish surgeon, Edward Canny Ryall, whose family seemed to have a tradition of setting up such hospitals, and who was said to have chosen this name because there were no saints' names left.

37. Kershaw, *Special Hospitals*, 62–4.

38. Information from *London Medical Directory* and *Medical Directory* of various years.

39. Frequently the development of hospitals is seen as medicine, or profession, propelled. The importance of patient demand should not be underestimated.

40. 'Hospital distress', *British Medical Journal*, no. 1 (1860), 458.

41. ibid.

42. ibid.

43. ibid.

44. ibid.

45. Op. cit., 459.

46. ibid.

47. ibid.

48. 'Annual meeting of the British Medical Association', *British Medical Journal*, no. 2 (1860), 627.

49. Op. cit., 628. There was great concern that charity was being 'abused' by those able to pay a GP for treatment. For charity abuse, see H. Burdett, *Hospitals and Asylums of the World*, 4 vols (1891–3); H. Burdett, *Cottage Hospitals, General, Fever, and Convalescent. Their Progress, Management, and Work in Great Britain and Ireland, and the United States of America*, 3rd edn (The Scientific Press, London 1896), 42.

50. 'Annual meeting of the British Medical Association', *British Medical Journal*, no. 2 (1860), 629.

51. *British Medical Journal*, no. 2 (1860), 582.

52. ibid.

53. 'A special hospital', *British Medical Journal*, no. 2 (1864), 582.

54. ibid.

55. C. Morson, *St Peter's Hospital for Stone* (S. Livingstone, Edinburgh and London, 1960), 15–17.

56. 'Mr Walter Coulson and the Hospital for Stone', *British Medical Journal*, no. 2 (1866), 703.

57. Op. cit., 704.

58. 'Note', *British Medical Journal*, no. 1 (1868), 561.

59. ibid.

60. Morson, *St Peter's Hospital*, 21.

61. 'Frederick Salmon', *Lancet*, no. 1 (1868), 68.

62. ibid.

63. 'Frederick Salmon', *British Medical Journal*, no. 1 (1868), 476.

64. Granshaw, *St Mark's Hospital*, 46–8, 73.

65. Op. cit., 51–2, 74.

66. Third Report from the Select Committee of the House of Lords on Metropolitan Hospitals, *British Parliamentary Papers*, 13 (1892), lix–lxvii.

67. *Plarr's Lives of the Fellows of the Royal College of Surgeons of England*, rev. by Sir D'Arcy Power with W.G. Spencer and G.E. Gask, 2 vols (pr. John Wright & Sons, Bristol, 1930). Continued as Sir D'Arcy Power and W.R. Le Fanu, *Lives of the Fellows of the Royal College of Surgeons of England, 1930–1951* (London, The Royal College of Surgeons, 1953).

68. 'Sir John Bland-Sutton (1855–1936)', *Plarr's Lives* (1953), 90.

69. ibid.

70. 'Sir Henry Butlin (1845–1912)', *Plarr's Lives* (1930), 178.

71. 'Percy Furnivall (1868–1938)', *Plarr's Lives* (1953), 311–12; Granshaw, *St Mark's Hospital*, 162–3, 172.

72. 'Robert Bickersteth (1787–1857)', *Plarr's Lives* (1930), 96; for Edinburgh, see G.B. Risse, *Hospital Life in Enlightenment Scotland.*

Care and Teaching at the Royal Infirmary of Edinburgh (Cambridge University Press, Cambridge, London, and New York, 1986).

73. 'Edward Bickersteth (1828–1908)', *Plarr's Lives* (1930), 95–6; C. Newman, *The Evolution of Medical Education in the Nineteenth Century* (Oxford University Press, London, 1957).

74. 'Robert Alexander Bickersteth (1862–1924)', *Plarr's Lives* (1930), 97.

75. See, for example, Granshaw, *St Mark's Hospital*, 108–9, 124–31.

76. Peterson, *Medical Profession*; Lawrence, 'Incommunicable knowledge'.

77. See, for example, R. Stevens, *Medical Practice in Modern England: The Impact of Specialisation and State Medicine* (Yale University Press, New Haven, 1966); Granshaw, *St Mark's Hospital*, 185–6.

78. C. Gordon-Watson, *Forty Years in Surgical Harness*, typescript, St Bartholomew's Hospital Medical College Library, 4–5.

79. Ruth Levitt, *The Reorganised National Health Service* (Croom Helm, London, 1979); Ruth Hodgkinson, *The Origins of the National Health Service: The Medical Service* (Wellcome Institute, London, 1967); John Pater, *The Origins of the National Health Service* (King's Fund Historical Series, London, 1981).

80. 'A new postgraduate centre?', *Lancet*, no. 2 (1961), 1,269.

9

From Friedenheim to hospice:
a century of cancer hospitals[1]

Caroline C.S. Murphy

Archaeological evidence shows that cancer, like the poor, has always been with us. Special cancer hospitals, however, are a far more recent phenomenon – though nothing like as new as the professional group of cancer specialists now known as oncologists.[2] Although the nineteenth-century origins of cancer hospitals may appear similar to those of other special hospitals, their emphasis on terminal care is more reminiscent of the hospice tradition of religious foundations. Unlike many of the other special hospitals, they did not primarily promote themselves as new centres for the development of scientific medicine. Plans made by the cancer hospitals in the 1890s for the establishment of 'hospices' – freed from any religious connotations under the name of 'Friedenheims' – illustrate recognition of the particular needs of the dying, though in the event they came to nothing. The competing demands for the support of clinical laboratory research into cancer were given priority, in the hope that discovery of a cure would remove the need for such 'Friedenheims'; this shift in emphasis has had lasting influence on provision for cancer and cancer patients.[3]

By the turn of the century, the pervasive influence of post-Bernardian scientific medicine effected a change in emphasis in the care offered by cancer hospitals. In the twentieth century they became centres for the development of surgical and radiotherapeutic treatments for cancer, while abandoning the medical treatments developed in the nineteenth century. The need for specialist care of the dying was eclipsed for three-quarters of a century, during which it was thought that the main priority in cancer was more research to uncover its uniquely obscure cause and thereby a cure. In the 1960s and 1970s the suffering of the dying, abandoned by the medical system, was given unprecedented publicity. The professional medical establishment had become geared to successful cures, and was seen to have lost the ability to cope with death. The hospice movement, operating in Britain independently of the NHS, put care of the dying firmly back on to the clinical agenda. Significantly, perhaps, the hospice movement does not yet appear to be aware of its stillborn precursor of a century ago.[4] This chapter cannot provide a comprehensive picture of the history of cancer hospitals; it does, however, hope to show how the demands of those dying of cancer have influenced the development of a very small group of special hospitals.

The Catholic religious tradition of provision of care for the sick and dying gave rise to the great charity hospitals of Britain, which fell into lay hands after the Reformation and the dissolution of the monastries. The establishment of scientific, rational medicine in the hands of licensed doctors and – in the aftermath of Florence Nightingale and her generation – professional nurses produced a change of emphasis in the way medicine was practised. Treatment of the patient with a view to curing a specific disease superseded the more traditional holistic approach to care of the body as the temporary vessel of the immortal soul. Having lost the support of the church, however, voluntary hospitals gained financial support on the basis of impressive statistics, preferably including few deaths. Excision of cancers has always been one of the more common forms of operative surgery, despite Hippocrates' admonition that the cancer patient would do better if left alone.[5] Although the histological nature of the variety of growths diagnosed as cancers in the past is now a matter of speculation, it is the case that 'cancer' patients were regularly admitted to the surgical wards of general hospitals.[6] At the same time, one of the devices used to 'massage' the hospital statistics was the exclusion from the wards of those with 'inoperable' cancers. This meant that there was no access to professional nursing care for those with advanced cancers who could not afford to pay.

Whatever doubts there may now be about the inaccurate diagnoses of leg ulcers, syphilitic sores, and mammary cysts as 'cancer', it is certain that by the late nineteenth century cancer had a reputation as being malign, painful, evil-smelling, and deadly. There were many theories of its cause, and plentiful 'quack' cures were available. The most consistent line adopted by the orthodox medical profession was that cancer could be cured with the knife if treated early enough. Just as long-standing as this surgical belief has been patients' fear of operations and the dread that the diagnosis 'cancer' meant certain and painful death.

With general hospitals unwilling to take in patients with advanced cancer, where were such patients to go and who was to treat them? The majority died at home in the care of their families, with scant help offered by GPs, who saw cancer only rarely during careers dominated by the treatment of contagious diseases. For those with large houses, secure incomes, and servants to change the linen and deal with the more distressing symptoms of the disease, this was manageable. Poor law infirmaries provided care for those accepted into the charge of the parish as paupers, but the 'respectable poor' faced the prospect that the diagnosis of cancer would break up families unable to provide adequate care. If it was the family breadwinner who was ill (often the case when the cancer was a direct result of industrial exposure to carcinogens), the whole family could be reduced to pauperism. The death of the head of the household in the poor law infirmary would then leave his bereaved family stigmatized as paupers.[7]

The inadequacy of the provision of treatment for those suffering from cancer meant that there was nowhere in the country where cancer (a disease taking many forms) could be studied. This was a fact that came home very forcibly to Dr William Marsden, the founder of London's Royal Free Hospital, when his wife died of cancer of the ovary in 1852. There was nothing that he could do for her while she was alive, but after her death he established a cancer hospital, which, like his general hospital, was also 'free' (no admission tickets were required). He hoped that by bringing a large number of cancer cases together, doctors specializing in the treatment of cancer would produce new, more effective, treatments. The hospital's basic role was to provide care until death; as a result, the small new hospital had a higher death rate than most of the larger established infirmaries. An early approach to Queen Victoria in search of patronage for the new hospital was turned down on the grounds that the disease was provided for in the general infirmaries. The first few annual reports produced by the hospital emphasized the preponderance of patients who had previously been turned away as 'untreatable' from such establishments. This evidence of the hospital's distinctive role was probably important in its eventual success in securing royal patronage.[8]

The London Cancer Hospital, now known as the Royal Marsden Hospital, was actually the second special cancer facility established in the capital. At the end of the eighteenth century, a cancer ward had been established at the Middlesex Hospital with money given by Samuel Whitbread. That cancer ward was established specifically for the care of the moribund – those with 'inoperable' cancer – who were excluded from care in the rest of the hospital and the rest of the London teaching hospitals.[9] The cancer ward had no imitators and produced few cancer specialists, though it was useful to the Middlesex Hospital in providing cancer patients for teaching the medical students about the then 'rare' disease. Care for the dying was a luxury that could only be afforded if there was a generous benefactor able to provide a large capital sum. As we shall see, Samuel Whitbread started a tradition of brewers supporting the care and treatment of cancer, a tradition that lapsed for some time after his death but was continued in the twentieth century.

While both the London Cancer Hospital and the Middlesex cancer ward offered care for the dying, only the Cancer Hospital produced its own medical 'cure' for cancer. William Marsden and his son Alexander developed the use of an 'arsenical mucillage' as a form of (reportedly painless) caustic which could be applied directly to a superficial tumour, causing it to slough off. This treatment, very much the product of a world in which the application of caustics, blisters, and leeches was the mainstay of practical medicine, did not enhance the standing of the Cancer Hospital.[10] At the Middlesex, the surgical tradition was perhaps too powerful to allow any such developments, though various medical treatments were tested on cancer ward patients – tests which in retrospect make very interesting reading.[11]

During the mid-nineteenth century, specialist hospitals based on the application of new scientific ideas and methods were proliferating in London. In developing the use of caustics, and continuing the traditional use of dangerously poisonous heavy metals, the Marsdens were not very 'progressive'. This did not mean that their hospital was without its imitators. Six years after its establishment, the Leeds Hospital for the Skin, Cancerous and Scrofulous Affections was opened, but only remained in operation for thirty-two years – the duration of its founder's career.

Granshaw has observed that in London most of the nineteenth-century specialist hospitals were established by medical men, while the eighteenth-century general hospitals had had lay origins.[12] The cancer hospitals founded in various British cities follow this pattern. Between 1857 and 1886, medical men in Leeds, Liverpool, Manchester, and Glasgow established cancer hospitals, all of which had failed by the outbreak of the Great War. Such failure was to be the fate of many nineteenth-century special hospitals on losing their founders. The cancer hospitals which failed did not act as proving-grounds for a specialty of cancer treatment. They were regarded by the medical profession as something far closer to 'quack' emporia where medical cure-alls were applied to superficial complaints of an uncertain nature. Medical cures for cancer were regarded as little more than wart charms, not as valuable contributions to scientific medicine.

The influence of surgeons on the development of cancer treatments is well illustrated by the experience of one of their number when he adopted a non-surgical method of treating cancer. Hugh Murray, who had worked as an assistant to Lister before receiving further training in Germany, established the Glasgow Cancer and Skin Institution in 1886. While Marsden claimed not to be competing with the established infirmaries, Murray specifically offered a medical alternative to the normal surgical treatment of cancer. Murray received no support from other Glasgow medical men who, it was reported, opposed him bitterly when he abandoned the knife for medical treatment. But he did have support from politically influential members of the citizenry in his regard for 'the knife treatment of cancer as the reproach and opprobrium of surgery'.[13] This support took the practical form of subscriptions when, in 1889, Dr Murray sought to expand his hospital. Unfortunately for Murray, some of his subscribers were those who supported the orthodox use of surgery in cancer. By 1893 they had replaced him as medical superintendant of 'his' hospital with an innovative surgeon, George Beatson. The Glasgow Cancer Hospital then took its place as a respected part of the Glasgow medical establishment – accepted as a place for surgical teaching – but it had problems attracting enough patients with 'true' cancer to be subjected to such surgery. Hugh Murray, on leaving the Glasgow Cancer Hospital, successfully ran his Glasgow Cancer and Skin Institution, for outpatients only.

The Glasgow Cancer Hospital did not remain unique as a cancer hospital recognized as a part of the local medical establishment. The Manchester Cancer Hospital was established adjacent to the Royal Infirmary by the executors of the Whitworth estate, under the chairmanship of a Manchester businessman, academic, and politician, Chancellor R.C. Christie.[14] In some ways, this hospital was very like the much larger London Cancer Hospital, providing for the care of the dying who were above the pauper class for whom the infirmary would not provide: unlike the London, however, it was not necessarily free. From the Hospital's foundation, it was intended to learn more about the nature of cancer in order to improve its treatment; the Hospital was immediately accepted as a useful addition to Manchester's hospital provision.

The London Cancer Hospital remained somewhat on the fringes of orthodox London medical practice at the end of the century, after the death of its founder William Marsden. One reason for this was the idiosyncratic (and high) profile of the hospital's consulting surgeon, Herbert Snow. Snow published extensively on the subject of cancer treatment and was a regular contributor to the correspondence columns of the *BMJ*.

In 1890 he published 'On the re-appearance (recurrence) of cancer after apparent extirpation, with suggestion for its prevention; and general remarks on the operative treatment of malignant growths', which was reviewed in the *BMJ* with his 'The palliative treatment of incurable cancer, with an appendix on the use of the opium pipe'.[15] The reviewer applauded Snow's advocacy of early excision as the best treatment for cancer and his belief in cancer as a 'local disease' rather than the product of heredity. Where the reviewer differed with him was in his attribution of 'too much influence on such conditions as mental distress and worry and general debility' as the causes of cancer. Snow had used opium in the relief of pain in cancer patients since 1876, because of his belief that the disease had neurotic origins; opium-smoking was *recommended* as a means of establishing an opium habit. In 1893 Snow combined the use of opium and cocaine for pain relief; he published his successful results in 1896.[16] His mixture formed the basis of the Brompton cocktail, which was to play such a large part in Cicely Saunders' establishment of hospice care for the dying about seventy years later. In the 1890s, though, it appears to have attracted little interest.

At this time, radical cancer surgery such as Halsted's radical mastectomy, oöphorectomy, and Wertheim's hysterectomy were becoming established parts of general surgical practice.[17] These operations could not be carried out in private houses; they became common in voluntary general hospitals. Those cancer hospitals which were not free were able to charge surgical patients for the use of 'pay beds' in rooms alongside their charity wards. The extra pressure that the increased use of radical surgery placed on the available beds was doubtless in some part responsible for the decision reached independently by the London, Manchester, and Glasgow cancer hospitals to establish 'Friedenheims'. A Friedenheim – a 'home of peace' for the dying – had been established for terminal TB patients in Germany in the 1880s (though the word never seems to have reached a German dictionary). The *Medical Directory*, however, shows that the first British Friedenheim, the Princess Alexandra's Friedenheim, was opened in Upper Avenue, Swiss Cottage (now the site of the Camden Local History Library) in 1889.[18]

The cancer hospitals in three of Britain's largest industrial cities planned to open such homes in the country, where their patients would go, not to convalesce, but to die in peace and comfort. While all three hospitals did increase their provision for surgical treatment, none of them ever opened a Friedenheim. As belief in the new, more aggressive surgery strengthened, and the methods of physiological research repeatedly proved their success in the control of infectious diseases, investment in homes for the hopeless seemed increasingly inappropriate. In 1902 the Imperial Cancer Research Fund (ICRF) was established in the belief that, given £½ million and twenty years, cancer would be cured as a result of the work of scientists in its laboratories.[19] The cancer hospitals, recognizing that research would attract greater support than the care of the dying, all shelved their Friedenheim plans and opened research laboratories.

Those cancer hospitals which adopted the new scientific approach to the disease tended to be those which survived into the twentieth century; those which were not able to adopt the new approach failed. There was one exception to this: St Catherine's Home for Cancer and Incurables in Bradford continued to provide a home for the dying well into the twentieth century. The Leeds Hospital for the Skin, Cancerous and Scrofulous Affections, the Manchester Hospital for the Skin, Cancer and Scrofula and All Chronic Diseases, and the Liverpool Tumour Hospital had all folded around 1889.[20] What remained of Hugh Murray's Glasgow Cancer and Skin Institution was to suffer directly from the influence of the ICRF.

In 1911 the Fund's Director, E.F. Bashford, included Murray as one of the cancer quacks castigated in his article 'Cancer, credulity and quackery' in the *British Medical Journal*.[21] Murray took no action concerning the article (he was old and died in 1914), but Dr Robert Bell of the Battersea Anti-Vivisection Hospital sued Bashford for libel over his description as a 'quack'. Bell was another surgeon who relinquished surgery, and was later to establish cancer wards for the dietetic and medicinal treatment of cancer. The court did not accept Bashford's argument that Bell's refusal to act on the result of mouse experiments and use surgery amounted to quackery, and Bashford was ordered to pay £2,000 damages.[22] After this courtroom defeat, Bashford did not remain in his position at the ICRF for long; he retired prematurely. Ironically, although Bashford's claim that surgery was the sole treatment for cancer was rejected by the court, the medical profession accepted that surgery should always be used as the first and main treatment for the disease, except in the case of superficial and skin cancers, for which a third alternative to the traditional choice of surgical or medical treatment became available.

Radiology and radiotherapy

X-rays were discovered at the end of 1895 and were first used in the treatment of cancer in 1896, though such early experiments in no way constituted an effective cancer treatment regime. Radioactivity was discovered in 1897 and radium in 1898: X-ray and radium therapy, however, took some time to become established as more than 'scientific' quack nostrums, fit only to be dismissed with such chemical nostrums as trypsin, arsenic, mercury, and potassium iodide.[23] The discovery of X-rays and their therapeutic use followed Finsen's successful development of ultraviolet light treatment in Denmark. UV was particularly useful in the treatment of skin diseases such as lupus (TB of the skin) and skin cancer. When it was established that X-rays, like UV, were constituents of health-giving sunlight, both forms of rays were used by dermatologists. The lead in this development in dermatology came from the London Hospital, which had benefited from an unwanted gift of a large UV treatment apparatus from Princess Alexandra in 1900.[24] The use of these different ray therapies in the treatment of skin cancer and other skin conditions continued the traditional association of cancer and skin which can be seen in the names of the nineteenth-century institutions. The accurate diagnosis of superficial cancers and their separation from non-cancerous conditions was a problem compounded by the tendency of syphilitic sores and leg ulcers to become 'malignant'. It was only with the development of reliable pathological techniques that accurate diagnosis and a specific definition of malignancy became possible.

From the time of their discovery, the main use of X-rays in medicine has been diagnostic. In those hospitals which had a medical electrician, this diagnostic work fell to him, leaving dermatologists such as James Sequira, at the London Hospital, to develop X-ray cancer treatments. In Manchester, X-ray treatments were successfully developed by the dermatologist at the Skin Hospital, where the Cancer Hospital sent appropriate patients. The Cancer Hospital found the technical difficulties of running their own X-ray plant too great to justify its use on the small number of patients involved at the small hospital.[25] In Glasgow, the medical electrician at the Royal Infirmary, Dr J. Macintyre (primarily an otolaryngologist), had an 'electric pavilion' before X-rays were discovered. He was so successful in his development of X-ray cancer treatments that no attempt was made to emulate him at the small Cancer Hospital down the road.[26] In all three cities, the cancer hospitals concentrated in the first decade of this century upon developing their research laboratories and their surgical facilities. These attracted patients who were not of the 'hospital class', as well as terminal charity cases, who were still turned away at the general infirmaries. Patients accommodated in 'home' beds until death accounted for a decreasing proportion of the work of the cancer hospitals. In Glasgow, a domiciliary service provided patients with, *inter alia*, coal, food, inflatable pillows, and clean bed linen, to ease dying at home. In the hospitals, the dying patients increasingly gave way to patients admitted for aggressive treatment aimed at cure; the treatment was often a combination of surgery and radiotherapy.

Radium (which was found to have a half-life of nearly 2,000 years) spontaneously produces the radioactive gas radon. For many years radon, rather than radium, the rarest and most valuable element in the world, was usually used for medical treatments. Radon gas, which was recommended for a vast range of conditions, was taken in a solution of water, directly inhaled, or sealed into tubes and implanted in body cavities. In the late 1890s naturally-occurring radon solutions were discovered to have been in use at spas for centuries before the discovery of radiation. The use of this discovery in advertising by both spas and industrial producers of radium products did not enhance the position of radium in the pharmacopoeia: Marie Curie's claim that it was a cancer specific did, however, increase patient demand for radium treatments.[27]

Gamma rays, like UV and X-rays, were found naturally in health-giving sunlight; they were regarded as natural and healthy like the other forms of physical therapy, such as electricity, heat, light, water, and massage. Radium institutes were established in most of the European capitals. It appears to have been King Edward VII who was directly responsible for the establishment of the London Radium Institute – Britain's first. He was himself successfully treated with radium (nearly 300 mg of salt were used), and he insisted that such treatment be available to his subjects. In both London and Manchester, brewers were the major supporters of outpatient radium institutes, which were, in a sense, radium dispensaries.[28] Just prior to the Great War, radium institutes were established in London and Manchester; radium supplies were also purchased for various cities around the UK, including Glasgow, Sheffield, Dublin, Plymouth, and Hull.

Although radium was rarely mentioned without reference to the belief that it might cure cancer, the majority of patients treated with radium before 1920 were suffering from arthritic and other chronic but not cancerous conditions. The only cancer hospital with more than a few milligrams of radium was the London Cancer Hospital, but new radium treatments were largely developed at the radium institutes, which increasingly specialized in cancer treatment.

After the Great War, the newly-formed Medical Research Council distributed radium for use in a multi-centre research scheme for the development of cancer treatments. The centres chosen were virtually all large general hospitals; only tiny amounts went for research to Lord Rutherford at the Cavendish Laboratories and to the London Radium Institute. Small amounts went to St Mark's and St Peter's, both of which had added 'cancer' to their titles before the outbreak of the war. The cancer hospitals were excluded from the scheme, apparently on the grounds that they were small – government radium would be in danger of being under-used. In the event, the radium was under-used in the large general hospitals which did receive it. One of these was the Middlesex Hospital, where the eighteenth-century cancer wards had been transformed from a charitable home for the dying into a centre for treatment and research.[29]

Despite the snub they received from the MRC, the small charitable institutions did not abandon cancer research and treatment, but terminal care became less important. In Manchester, the Radium Institute successfully developed a treatment regime for cancer of the mouth and throat. Working in co-operation with the nearby cancer hospital, they were able to develop inpatient treatments. Patients receiving these treatments tended to take beds which would previously have been used for terminal care, a change which was not universally welcomed by those on the hospital board. The poor law infirmaries had improved considerably in the first thirty years of the twentieth century, but they certainly did not provide ideal care for terminal cancer patients.[30]

During the economic stringencies of the 1920s and 1930s there was little money available for the expansion of the cancer hospitals, but there were demands for an increased radium supply, especially after the success of the MRC scheme. Until the mid-1920s, radiation was often only recommended as a palliative in those cases where surgery had failed. Primary radiation therapy could only be developed on those patients who adamantly refused surgery.[31] During the 1920s successive falls in the price of radium made it an increasingly popular object of medical patronage. By the end of the 1920s hospitals – large and small, all over the country – were seeking to secure their own supplies for cancer treatments.

Cancer therapy or radiotherapy

After a radium census in 1929, a national radium supply was purchased, to avert the consequences of virtually every hospital having its own inadequately-managed, extremely dangerous radium. A National Radium Trust, acting through a National Radium Commission, supplied radium to a series of National Radium Centres. Each centre was based on a teaching hospital and a university physics department; cancer hospitals were not even considered when the structure was drawn up. The only national radium centres to include pre-existing radium institutes and/or cancer hospitals were at Manchester and Liverpool. In London, which did not have to follow this pattern of regional centres – in deference to the anarchic free-for-all between the competing teaching hospitals – the Cancer Hospital was by no means the pre-eminent centre for radiotherapy. Bart's, the Middlesex, and the Westminster fought for this distinction; at the Cancer Hospital radiotherapy received scant regard, but it did benefit from the increased supplies of radium.[32]

Increased confidence that radium offered a cure for cancer is shown by the Mount Vernon Hospital's decision to change from a TB sanatorium to a specialist radiotherapeutic cancer hospital. Another cancer hospital established in London during the early 1920s was the Marie Curie Cancer Hospital, staffed by women for the treatment of women cancer patients.[33] This hospital was a particularly successful participant in the MRC radium research scheme, developing the first successful treatment for cancer of the uterus. These two new cancer hospitals were like almost all the other remaining cancer hospitals – centres for the development of radium therapy. Even the relatively small Glasgow Cancer Hospital opened its own radium institute; the emphasis of the hospital had changed from care of the dying to radical aggressive surgery and radiotherapy.[34]

The success of the new cancer treatments based on the integration of surgery and radium therapy was demonstrated in the terms of the 1939 Cancer Act. This established a financial structure for the provision of radium treatments for cancer patients throughout the country. This structure was needed despite a fall in the price of radium (as Canadian radium came on the market), because high-energy radiation-beam therapies became established in the late 1930s.[35]

In 1939 the Second World War intervened, preventing the implementation of the Cancer Act, whose provisions were superseded by those of the National Health Service Act of 1946. Much to the regret of many involved with it, this brought an end to the National Radium Commission; there would no longer be an independent body monitoring and controlling the medical use of radionucleides.[36] By this time, radium was beginning to be replaced by radio-cobalt and iridium, isotopes which did not continually produce a dangerous radioactive gas like the radon produced by radium. Under the NHS, most cancer hospitals lost their 'special' designation and were gradually integrated into large general hospitals. Radiotherapy became a regional specialty which, like plastic surgery, was to be made available at one site – usually a general teaching hospital – within every region.

Significantly, the discussions concerning the possibility of a role for the NRC in the NHS had centred on the question of the extent to which radiotherapy could be regarded as 'cancer therapy'. It was tempting before the Second World War to present radiotherapy as the cancer therapy applicable wherever surgery could not offer a cure. This was not the full story, though. Radiotherapy was also used to treat some non-malignant conditions, and some practitioners were worried that, if radiotherapy were only presented as cancer therapy, some patients would avoid treatment for fear of stigma. There were also some forms of cancer which neither surgery nor radiotherapy could hope to cure.

In the wake of the Second World War, the medicinal treatment of cancer was reintroduced. The aggressive cancer chemotherapeutic use of nitrogen mustards and their derivatives were actually a direct consequence of a military accident, but the new antibiotics and synthetic hormones helped to open up new potential aggressive treatments aimed at cure.[37] This made sense of the location of cancer patients in large general hospitals where teams of surgeons, physicians, and radiotherapists could develop appropriate courses of treatment for their patients. Terminal care was not, however, regarded as a specialty, and no special provision was made for the dying. Part of the reason for this can be seen in the speech Bevan made on presenting the NHS Bill to Parliament. He described how he 'would rather be kept alive in the efficient if cold altruism of a large hospital than expire in a gush of warm sympathy in a small one'.[38] That is all very well where there is the prospect of recovery. The health service he created had little room for the dying – the embarrassing evidence of the failure of medicine to make man immortal. His despised 'gush of warm sympathy' was missed, once reorganization and rebuilding had done away with the small hospitals (especially the cottage hospitals). During the first twenty years of the NHS, it became increasingly common for people to die in hospital, on general wards, away from the support of their families, under the care of medical staff ill-equipped to cope with death.[39]

The hospice reborn

In the white heat of the technological revolution of the 1960s, death came to be seen as the great 'medical failure' rather than a natural part of life, to be coped with rather than ignored. New, more aggressive cancer treatments were developed which left patients and relatives wondering whether the treatment was worse than the disease and demanding an answer to the difficult question 'Is a few more weeks of life worth the pain and suffering involved?' This was a question which did not attract strong charitable support from the ICRF or the Cancer Research Campaign, the latter a charity originally conceived as a means of routing money into clinical rather than laboratory research. Research into care for the dying attracted little support from the existing charities. A new cancer charity, the Marie Curie Cancer Relief Fund, was established; this supported home care for the terminally ill.[40] The area which needed most attention – and appeared most intractable – was pain control. Successful research into this problem was carried out, not in a teaching hospital, but in a South London hospice, run by nuns who devoted themselves to easing their patients' passage from the world of the living to that of the dead.

Stoddard, in her book *The Hospice Movement: A Better Way of Dying*, traces the origins of the modern hospice movement to the Dublin Hospice, established by Sister Mary Aikenhead, a Sister of Charity, who had been a co-worker and contemporary of Florence Nightingale.[41] In 1902, the English Sisters of Charity opened St Joseph's Hospice in London; by this time there were already several homes for the dying, including the Hostel of God (founded in 1892, now the Trinity Hospice), St Luke's Hospital (a 'home for the dying poor', founded in 1893, now Hereford Lodge) and the Friedenheim Hospital (founded 1892). Unlike the religious establishments, the Friedenheim Hospital, which later became the Princess Alexandra Friedenheim, is not mentioned in the work of the chroniclers of the hospice movement. 'Friedenheim' was, however, the title chosen by those who wanted to establish homes for the dying attached to new cancer hospitals in the 1890s.[42]

Research into the control of terminal cancer pain started at St Luke's Hospital in 1948, and was developed at St Joseph's Hospice between 1958 and 1965 by Cicely (now Dame Cicely) Saunders – one of those rare creatures, a doctor of medicine who is also qualified as a nurse (and almoner). This work would not have been possible in the USA, because of its dependence on the controlled use of heroin and cocaine, neither legal – even in medical use – in the USA. The value of the combination of these drugs had been established at the London Cancer Hospital by the surgeon Henry Snow. Snow's 'Brompton cocktail' (as the heroin and cocaine mixture was known) was far better received than his controversial observation that cancer was stress-related. This claim had attracted considerable criticism in the pages of the *BMJ*. The problem with terminal pain control, however, was to ensure that the patient was not simply caught on a seesaw between drug-induced oblivion and overwhelming pain. The objective was to keep the patient in a mental condition adequate to continue sharing life, even if only from bed, with family and friends. Cicely Saunders combined the 'Brompton cocktail' of heroin (or morphine) and cocaine in controlled doses with synthetic steroids, anti-inflammatories, cancer chemotherapy, and palliative radiotherapy.[43] The discovery that pain control was possible, though by no means simple, brought about what was possibly the greatest revolution in cancer treatment since the introduction of radium treatments.

In 1967, Dame Cicely Saunders, by now the personification of the hospice movement, established St Christopher's Hospice as the first research and teaching hospice. Her intention was to lay the scientific foundations of terminal care and in so doing make the care of the dying medically respectable. From 1969 St Christopher's ran a domiciliary care service, much like that run by the Glasgow Cancer Hospital before the First World War. In 1974, eighty years after its plan for a Friedenheim was shelved, the Royal Marsden opened a ward – the Horder Ward – to provide specialized care for the dying. From 1975, money became available from the National Society for Cancer Relief for the building of twenty-five-bed terminal-care centres on NHS land. By the mid-1980s the hospice movement has developed so far that it has now declared its aim to be not the provision of hospice beds for all moribund patients, but to have such an effect on attitudes and training that 'no dying patients, anywhere, should fail to find staff with sufficient awareness of their needs either to give help themselves or to call in others where they cannot do so'.[44] The NMTBD ('no more to be done') that was regularly written on the notes of patients failed by radiotherapy should become a thing of the past.

Ironically, it was during this minor revolution in cancer care that Britain's first Friedenheim was closed in bizarre circumstances. In 1958, after staffing difficulties, the 120-year-old buildings of the St Columba's Hospital, as it was called by then, were demolished to make way for the Civic Centre at Swiss Cottage.[45] At this point, St Columba's, which was described by Sir John Fremantle as 'an old voluntary hospital with a remarkably fine atmosphere', was not under threat of closure, though the number of beds was

halved to thirty-five.[46] The building it moved to, The Elms
on Spaniard's Lane, was said to be the second largest house
in London (after Buckingham Palace), but it had no bed lift
– so the upper floors went unused. In 1979 the Kensington,
Chelsea, and Westminster Area Health Authority started
trying to close it, with a view to saving about £200,000 per
year and to realize capital on the sale of the site. At the end
of 1980 the NUPE campaign against the closure of the
twenty-seven-bed hospital for terminally-ill cancer patients
had extended from negotiations with various statutory bodies
to a picketing and leafleting campaign, including a picket of
the TUC Annual Conference. The Health Authority, in its
desire to clear the site, started transferring patients in private
ambulances.[47] After a union official had been injured by one
of these vehicles – and a patient had died in transit – one
driver decided that he could not take the remaining dying
man from his ward. For the first few weeks of 1981, while the
hospice movement was gaining support throughout the world
for specialized supportive care for the dying, one old man lay
dying with his London hospice (one of only seven then run
by the NHS) dying around him on its spectacular 7-acre site,
overlooking the vale where Keats heard his nightingale.[48]
After his death, proposals that The Elms should become a
test-tube baby clinic, an American hospital, or be converted
into flats came to nothing. The building was sold to an Arab
for £2.6 million, but remains unoccupied because of planning
problems over a proposed conversion of the stable block into
a harem.[49]

The London Cancer Hospital had by then established its
specialized ward for terminal care; it had developed its own
proposed Friedenheim site (in Sutton) as a modern cancer
hospital many years previously. The house which had been
offered to the Glasgow Cancer Hospital as a Friedenheim had
burnt down before it was equipped to receive patients, but in
the late 1970s its grounds provided the site for the new Beatson Cancer Research Laboratories when they outgrew the old
Glasgow Cancer Hospital. The foundations of the old
building are now grassed over, overlooked by the veterinary
school, where AIDS vaccines are being developed. We live in
the remains of our history, just as much in the field of cancer
treatment as elsewhere. The demands for terminal care were
never pushed out by the putative success of research into the

cause of cancer. What may seem rather ironic is the way in which palliative care has come to regain the respectability it lost from the 1940s to the 1960s.

When Beatson took over the Glasgow Cancer Hospital from the unorthodox Hugh Murray in the 1890s, he gained international acclaim for his introduction of the ovariectomy as a treatment for breast cancer in pre-menopausal women. After the deaths of all the patients with whom he had had impressive results for several years, he wrote a disclaimer of this 'cure for cancer'. He could not recommend it; it was only palliative. When artificial female hormones became available, they were used to produce 'premature menopause' in much the same way that Beatson had brought it about surgically. When radium implants were first developed, they were only recommended as palliatives, to be used for the relief of local pain and symptoms. The 'real' treatment was surgery. One of the important elements of modern terminal care is, once again, palliative radiotherapy. It is reasonable to speculate that by the end of this century therapeutic spa treatments using radioactive muds and waters will have been reintroduced from the continent as part of the complete care of the cancer patient.

This may only be speculation, but it is certain that while general hospitals have extended the treatments they offer to cancer patients, the role of the special cancer hospital has in some important respects come full circle – from terminal care to aggressive treatment and back to terminal care – in the course of a century. If the lessons learned by hospices can be successfully introduced into general hospital practice, it will be in a sense a re-run of the passage of radiotherapy from special cancer hospitals into the general hospitals. This illustrates how small specialist centres have developed in the past and can still develop new aspects of patient care that may then usefully be taken up into more general use by the large institutions.

Notes

1. Dr Murphy is now the Education Officer (Ethics) of the Royal Society for the Prevention of Cruelty to Animals. This work was financed by the Wellcome Trust through a post-doctoral Fellowship

and postgraduate scholarship and by the Science and Education Research Council – Social Science Research Council joint committee postgraduate scholarship.

2. M.B. Shimkin, *Contrary to Nature* (US Department of Health, Education, and Welfare Public Health Services, National Institute of Health, Washington, 1977), 19–20. J. Austoker, 'Cancer research left to charity', *New Scientist*, no. 1,582 (1987), 28–9 and *A History of the Imperial Cancer Research Fund 1902 to 1986* (Oxford University Press, 1987).

3. C.C.S. Murphy, 'A history of radiotherapy to 1950: cancer and radiotherapy in Britain 1850–1950', PhD thesis, University of Manchester Institute of Science and Technology (1986), *passim*.

4. D. Winn, *The Hospice Way* (Macdonald, London, 1987), 23–4; S. Stoddard, *The Hospice Movement: A Better Way of Caring for the Dying* (Jonathan Cape, London, 1979) *passim*; and C. Saunders, D. Summers, and N. Teller (eds), *Hospice: the Living Idea* (Edward Arnold, London, 1981), *passim*.

5. Shimkin, *Contrary to Nature*, 24. In G.E.R. Lloyd, *Hippocratic Writings* (Penguin, London, 1978), 230, this aphorism – section VI, number 38 – is translated as 'It is better not to treat those who have internal cancers since, if treated, they die quickly; but if not treated they last a long time.'

6. G.B. Risse, *Hospital Life in Enlightenment Scotland: Care and Teaching at the Royal Infirmary Edinburgh* (Cambridge University Press, Cambridge, 1986), 164–6.

7. J. Woodward, *To Do The Sick No Harm: A Study of the British Voluntary Hospital System to 1875* (Routledge & Kegan Paul, London, 1974), 51 and 134. See also Murphy, 'History of Radiotherapy', 1.1–1.12.

8. F. Sandwith, *Surgeon Compassionate: The Story of Dr William Marsden* (Peter Davies, London, 1960), 193–261.

9. E. Wilson, *The History of the Middlesex Hospital* (Churchill, London, 1845), 17.

10. A. Marsden, *A New and Successful Mode of Treating Certain Forms of Cancer* (J. Churchill, London, 1869).

11. Minutes of the Cancer Investigation Committee of the Middlesex Hospital, 24 May 1904. See also J.W.G. Myler, 'Some empirical methods adopted in the treatment of inoperable cancer and their results', *Archives of the Middlesex Hospital*, vol. 2, March (1904), 65.

12. L. Granshaw, *St Mark's Hospital, London: A Social History of a Specialist Hospital* (King's Fund Historical Series, London, 1985), 6.

13. *The Glasgow Cancer and Skin Institution Annual Report* (1891), 11. See also G.T. Beatson (Sir), *A Short History of the Glasgow Royal Cancer Hospital* (The Glasgow Royal Cancer Hospital, 1930), 1.

14. T. Macdonald, 'Christie Hospital and Holt Radium Institute: foundation, development and achievements 1892–1962', M.Sc. thesis, University of Manchester Institute of Science and

Technology (1977).

15. H. Snow, 'On the re-appearance (recurrence) of cancer after apparent extirpation, with suggestions for its prevention; and general remarks on the operative treatment of malignant growths' and 'The palliative treatment of incurable cancer, with an appendix on the use of the opium pipe', *British Medical Journal*, vol. 2 (1890), 689–90.

16. H. Snow, 'Opium and cocaine in the treatment of cancerous disease', *British Medical Journal*, vol. 2 (1896), 718.

17. Murphy, 'History of radiotherapy', 1.23–1.28.

18. See the *Medical Directory* 1894–1913 under London: Special Hospitals.

19. Anon (probably J. Craigie), *Imperial Cancer Research Fund 1902–1952: Fifty Years of Cancer Research* (supplement to ICRF Annual Report, 1952), and C.E. Dukes, 'The origins and early history of the Imperial Cancer Research Fund', *Annals of the Royal College of Surgeons*, vol. 36 (1965), 325–9.

20. Information from various editions of the *Medical Directory* and from the area health authorities.

21. E.F. Bashford, 'Cancer, credulity and quackery', *British Medical Journal*, vol. 1 (1911), 1,221–30.

22. R. Bell, *Reminiscences of an Old Physician* (John Murray, London, 1924), 241–4 and Appendix. See also Medico Legal, 'Bell *v.* Bashford and the British Medical Association', *British Medical Journal*, vol. 1 (1912), 1,403–7 and 1,461–7.

23. Murphy, 'History of radiotherapy', 3.31–3.42. See also L.D. Longo, 'Electrotherapy in gynaecology: the American experience', *Bulletin of the History of Medicine*, vol. 60, no. 3 (1986), 340–66.

24. M. Rowbottom and C. Susskind, *Electricity and Medicine: History of Their Interaction* (San Francisco Press, 1984), 229–33. See also A.E. Clark-Kennedy, *The London: A Study in the Voluntary Hospital System 1740–1948* (Pitman Medical Publishing, London, 1963), 142–3. This equipment is on display in the Wellcome Galleries at the Science Museum, London.

25. Murphy, 'History of radiotherapy', 3.26.

26. A.L. Goodall, 'John Macintyre, pioneer radiologist 1857–1928', *Surgo*, Whitsun (1958), 119–26.

27. R. Reid, *Marie Curie* (Collins, London, 1974), 126, 133, and 224.

28. Murphy, 'History of radiotherapy', 3.43–3.63.

29. Op. cit., 5.1–5.14.

30. J.V. Pickstone, *Medicine and Industrial Society: A History of Hospital Development in Manchester and its Region, 1752–1946* (Manchester University Press, 1985), 256–64; G.E. Birkett, *Radium Therapy: Principles and Practice* (Cassell, London, 1931).

31. G.L. Keynes, *The Gates of Memory* (Oxford University Press, 1983), 211–16.

32. F.G. Spear and K. Griffiths, *The Radium Commission: A Short*

History of its Origins and Work 1929–1948 (HMSO, London, 1951).

33. Murphy, 'History of radiotherapy', 5.25–5.30.

34. Beatson, *Glasgow Royal Cancer Hospital* 7–9.

35. E.R. Landa, 'The first nuclear industry', *Scientific American*, vol. 247 (1982), 154–63.

36. Murphy, 'History of radiotherapy', 7.55–7.61.

37. G.B. Infield, *Disaster at Bari* (Hale, London, 1974), *passim*.

38. B. Abel-Smith, *The Hospitals 1800–1948: A Study in Social Administration in England and Wales* (Heinemann, London, 1964), 481.

39. Marie Curie Memorial Foundation, *Report on a National Survey Concerning Patients Nursed at Home* (Marie Curie Memorial Foundation, London, 1952), *passim*; and H.L.G. Hughes, *Peace at the Last – A Survey of Terminal Care in the United Kingdom* (The Calouste Gulbenkian Foundation, London, 1960), *passim*.

40. B.J. Lunt, *Terminal Cancer Care: Specialist Services Available in Great Britain in 1980* (Wessex Regional Cancer Organization, Southampton, 1980).

41. Stoddard, *The Hospice Movement*, 65.

42. Murphy, 'History of radiotherapy', 1.39–1.40.

43. R.G. Twycross, 'Relief of pain' in C. Saunders (ed.), *The Management of Terminal Malignant Disease* (Edward Arnold, London, 1984), 82–3.

44. C. Saunders, 'Evolution in terminal care' in Saunders (ed.), *Management of Terminal Malignant Disease*, 216.

45. *Hampstead and Highgate Express*, 11 July 1958.

46. *Hampstead and Highgate Express*, 14 Oct. 1955; see also *Hampstead and Highgate Express*, 14 Dec. 1979, 29 Aug., 24 Oct., 19 Sept., and 7 Nov. 1980.

47. *Morning Star*, 22 Oct. 1980.

48. *Hampstead and Highgate Express*, 21 Nov. 1980.

49. *Hampstead and Highgate Express*, 9 Nov. 1981; *Daily Telegraph*, 3 Dec. 1981. These newspaper cuttings are part of the special collection about St Columba's in the Camden Local History Library.

10

Managing medicine: creating a profession of hospital administration in the United States, 1895 – 1915

Morris J. Vogel

Hospitals are among the most complex of modern social institutions. They have assumed responsibility for the care of individuals confronting extreme crises. They mobilize some of society's most advanced intellectual and technological resources, and command substantial and growing proportions of the common wealth. And they are directed through formal bureaucratic structures and sophisticated management techniques that befit their roles and resources.

It is difficult to recall that not much more than a century ago hospitals did little more than provide settings in which physicians practised a minimally interventionist medicine on the small minority of the sick and injured who sought institutional treatment. Concentrated as they were in larger urban centres, the nation's few hospitals were outside the experience and even the imagination of most Americans. Furnishing room, board, and attention primarily to the socially marginal, hospitals were themselves marginal, little more than homes for the sick homeless. They furnished no special medical technologies, no therapies not otherwise available in the ordinary patient's home.[1]

The hospital was like the home in its informal administration as well. Though physicians increasingly involved themselves in determining institutional priorities, major decisions remained in the hands of lay trustees, the charitably-inclined individuals whose benefactions underwrote institutional expenses but whose primary responsibilities were focused elsewhere. The authority of hospital superintendents and the other managers who directed day-to-day operations rarely extended beyond control of the domestic staff and the purchase of food, coal, and other household provisions.

The American general hospital began to assume its modern form and significance at the turn of the twentieth century. The hundred or so institutions of the early 1870s grew to around 4,000 by 1910. By that date, towns of 10,000 residents might reasonably expect to have hospitals within their limits or nearby, and hospitals were regularly admitting middle-class patients who, a generation earlier, would have spurned their services.[2] Physicians had begun to reorganize their practices around the institution and the skilled nursing, laboratories, specialized facilities, and newly-developing medical technologies it offered. Patients were now more likely to be hospitalized for episodes of acute illness than for chronic care or recuperation, and their treatment was correspondingly more active and interventionist. Costs, as a consequence, were rising dramatically and in many cases outstripping the resources of private charity. The transformed institution could no longer be managed as informally as its predecessor.[3]

It was against this backdrop that the Association of Hospital Superintendents of the United States and Canada (which changed its name in 1906 to the American Hospital Association) first met in 1899. Eight superintendents – all but one from Cleveland, where the group met, and Detroit – and a publisher, whom the group elected to honorary membership, convened for two days in September to draft a charter for a national organization that would bring superintendents together regularly for the interchange of ideas about hospital management.[4]

The involvement of Del Sutton, the publisher, suggests that the organization was not a fore-ordained necessity. Sutton, who had been campaigning for a superintendent's group since he had begun *The National Hospital Sanitarium Record* in 1897, had a financial stake in creating the Association. Sutton intended his new journal as an advertising vehicle for suppliers to the growing hospital market. He had begun with a special relationship with the makers of Imperial Granum Food, a processed wheat food for convalescents, before the Association's charter meeting adopted his *Record* as its official organ. In his formal address to the second meeting in 1900, Sutton revealed something of his interest in the hospital market. Noting that the previous three years had seen the founding of 1,000 new hospitals, Sutton pointed out that vast sums were now spent in building and supplying hospitals. The *Record* published abbreviated accounts of Association proceedings for three years before the Association undertook this task itself in 1902. Sutton's journal survived until 1915, changing its name several times before it was purchased by the Association and discontinued in favour of the Association's newly-established *The Modern Hospital*.[5]

While Sutton had his own agenda in promoting the Association, he and the small group at the first meeting had struck a responsive chord. Thirty-one superintendents attended the 1900 meeting, forty-seven came in 1901, and more than 100 registered for the fourth meeting in 1902. By its tenth meeting in 1908, the new association had more than 450 members from across the United States and Canada.[6] These men and women joined together for a variety of reasons. The superintendents resembled other groups of Americans – managers, professionals, and the like – in new, rapidly growing, or evolving fields who affiliated with one another in new organizations to seek common answers to common problems, fellowship with others similarly situated, and ways of enhancing their status and self-esteem.[7]

The first generations of hospital superintendents had not been selected for their presumed technical competencies; indeed, they were meant to learn their craft on the job. Presiding over essentially domestic arrangements, the early nineteenth-century superintendent's chief qualifications had been his probity and his willingness to spend his life within the confining walls of the hospital. It is little wonder that retired ships' captains – men who had assumed responsibility for the fortunes of others – were heavily represented among *ante-bellum* stewards and superintendents. The role was that of a caretaker; superintendents were not expected to initiate or innovate.[8]

By the end of the nineteenth century, hospital superintendents had generally changed little in background and training from their predecessors. To be sure, a significant proportion of superintendents were now women, matrons or head nurses with responsibility for predominantly smaller hospitals, or religious superiors in charge of Catholic institutions. These women resembled their male counterparts in that they were chiefly qualified by virtue of being presumed satisfactory caretakers. But the radical transformation of the hospital then underway posed new challenges and created new opportunities and roles for superintendents.

Among the larger hospitals particularly – where change was likely to be most dramatic – superintendents had begun to look to each other informally for advice by the close of the nineteenth century. Circular letters had inquired about such newly-pressing issues as facilities for middle-class patients or whether physicians were permitted to charge fees for inpatient care. Superintendents had also started to tour other institutions – with the Massachusetts General and the new Johns Hopkins as favourite destinations – to familiarize themselves with the state of the managerial art. Superintendents from several Boston hospitals had met informally to discuss common concerns, and in New York City an on-going hospital conference brought together representatives of forty institutions.[9] The annual meetings of the American Hospital Association extended and institutionalized these informal practices. Formal papers, scheduled discussions, and face-to-face contact allowed superintendents to share the specialized knowledge of their craft and to seek guidance on subjects they found puzzling. Furnishing occasions for the exchange of institutional and personal experience, the new association and its regularly scheduled meetings made superintendents part of a national movement and fit their concerns into the early twentieth-century campaign for scientific management.[10]

Much of the discussion addressed the modernization of the hospital. Whether superintendents actively directed their institutions or merely gathered information for their trustees, they had to consider a broad range of new issues. Asepsis and the other demands of scientific medicine required, for example, that many older buildings be modified or replaced, and that the design of new structures accommodate current technologies. In many cases, superintendents found that they could no longer simply manage inherited physical plants, but they had to represent their institutions in architectural collaborations that balanced the needs of physicians and the financial resources of the institution.[11] The growing clinical orientation of medical education likewise imposed demands on hospitals, sometimes requiring superintendents to weigh the competing needs of medical staff, patient care, and teaching, and make appropriate recommendations to trustees.[12]

The aspect of the hospital's transformation in which the superintendent figured most conspicuously was the cost squeeze. Mounting expenses forced the modernizing hospital to look beyond the charity of its narrow circle of traditional donors. No longer could it rely as completely on informal appeals spearheaded by trustees. The fact that hospitals were attracting increasing numbers of middle-class patients expanded the possibility for financial support. By the early twentieth century, organized fund drives – in which superintendents co-operated with professional managers – were appealing to a broadened base of community support.[13]

But it was especially with their individual payments for patient care that the middle classes came to take on the burden of hospital funding. The hospitalization of the middle classes changed the nature of the traditional institution as fundamentally as scientific medicine. And superintendents took on much of the burden for fashioning the hospital's response to this growing patient class. Doctors bore the primary responsibility for attracting these paying patients through referrals, but it was largely left to domestic and nursing staffs under the superintendent's direction to adjust the day-to-day life of institutions originally intended for the poor to the care of middle-class patients and the recognition of their needs. Superintendents also had to implement cost accounting procedures to determine to what extent hospitals were subsidizing or profiting from paying patients.[14] At the same time, superintendents – much more than physicians – were expected to defend the interests of the hospital's original constituency of poor patients, whose care was coming now more often to be thought a drain on funds rather than the sacred duty it had been a half-century before.[15] Strains in the historic obligation to provide charitable care for the poor were evident, for example, in the obsessive concern with medical abuse. The accusation that patients who could afford to pay imposed on hospital charity by seeking free treatment had been heard before, but it acquired special urgency as middle-class patients began to seek hospital treatment and hospitals came to depend on their fees. Association meetings regularly featured papers demonstrating the pervasiveness of this practice and presenting stratagems to limit it.[16]

One is struck by the apparent trivia often exchanged under Association auspices. Some details seem to be no more than housekeeping hints. But even much of this mundane detail was motivated – and perhaps even necessitated – by the changing nature of the hospital. Superintendents wanting to remain current about techniques for maintaining asepsis, for example, had to concern themselves with flooring materials installed in operating rooms and with the way wards were swept. Hospitals competing for middle-class patients had to serve meals attractive to middle-class palates. And given the steeply-mounting expenses of the modernizing hospital, it is understandable that prudent administrators would also consider domestic economies.[17] J.T. Duryea, general medical superintendent of hospitals in Brooklyn, New York, struck perhaps the Association's keynote in his presidential address to the fourth annual convention. Arguing that superintendents could learn from each other's methods in managing the myriad details of their complex institutions, he declaimed, 'Show us how you keep your census high and your cost per diem low.'[18]

Association sessions were extraordinarily earnest in their consideration of such details of domestic management as the proper temperature to store lemons, how to mark sheets, and the importance of buying only foods in season. Underlying much of this concern was the effort to reduce expenses. Session after session added to the array of cost-cutting techniques: superintendents explained how to clean and re-use soiled gauze (furnishing softer and more absorbent bandages in the bargain); and how they confronted surgeons with comparative counts of instruments used (and therefore needing costly cleaning and sterilization) in operations.[19] The obsessive commitment of some turn-of-the-century superintendents to exaggerated and almost ludicrous economies must be understood as more than simple efforts to keep expenditures in check. Association activists should be recognized as ideologues, converts to the doctrine of efficiency then gaining broad social currency.

Superintendents joining together in the Association shared a sense of their mutual cause. Running through their early deliberations was the notion that they confronted common problems and would therefore profit by looking beyond their local communities and their personal experiences. It made little sense for an individual administrator to develop a solution to a problem that had already been resolved elsewhere. But the point of these meetings was not merely the exchange of information, important as that was. In their frequent reiteration of the complaint that they too often had to rely on their own judgement, superintendents made clear that they were searching for a body of objectifiable data, of certifiable knowledge.[20] The 'facts' of an administrative science would not only aid decision-making, but would also serve as the base of specialized knowledge on which superintendents could establish their claims to professional expertise. A seeming jumble of simple domestic wisdom, basic administrative procedure, construction technology, organizational schemes, customer relations, and professional aspiration was at its core an effort to work out a system of managerial science addressed to the special problems of the modern hospital. In this regard, as in their commitment to a cost-cutting efficiency, superintendents were full participants in the scientific management crusade of the early twentieth century.[21]

Like self-consciously scientific managers and technical experts in other fields, superintendents sought to forge a professional identity. A collective organization was an important strategy in this regard; meetings, journals, management handbooks, and courses of study offered more than an opportunity to share technique. The very fact that the superintendents developed a specialized organization at whose meetings they devoted themselves to the pursuit of arcane knowledge and worthy public ends signalled professionalism. Joining together allowed hospital administrators to define the special competencies required for the practice of their craft and to certify mutually that Association members were expert in the enterprise of hospital superintendency.[22] Within its first decade, the Association had developed standards for membership which, while generously inclusive, required that applicants be voted into fellowship in the Society. The appearance of organizations promoting and staking public claims about the expertise of their members and the public good they served was a salient characteristic of turn-of-the-century America. Following the lead of engineers, social scientists, and – most conspicuously – physicians, hospital administrators sought to capitalize on the authority American society increasingly granted those professing technical expertise.[23]

While discussions at early Association meetings generally proceeded from a widespread consensus that it was desirable to enhance the status and authority of superintendents, papers and recorded debates revealed less unanimity on specific agendas to meet these goals. For one thing, turn-of-the-century administrators came from a variety of backgrounds. A small but significant minority – some of whom directed the large and important urban hospitals – were physicians. Relatively secure in their credentials, they emphasized the importance of medical qualifications in carrying out administrative tasks. Male lay superintendents, on the other hand, tended to regard the business sense that had commended them to like-minded trustees as the most important skill for the roles they already had and for the increased authority most prized.[24] These men generally took the lead in Association discussions that treated the household arrangements at the core of early twentieth-century hospital administration as subjects for technical management analyses.[25] Management science may have been doubly attractive to these male lay superintendents because it offered the possibility of escaping the stigma of tasks broadly defined as feminine – a fact that could hardly go unnoticed in a field, many of whose practitioners were women. Women superintendents – a near majority at most early meetings – on the whole absented themselves from recorded discussions about exercising or augmenting the institutional power of the superintendency. This last fact may owe to internalized social and cultural constraints about appropriate public postures for women. The apparent reluctance to discuss power may stem equally from the specific institutional settings in which most women superintendents worked. Concentrated in smaller hospitals, they presided over comparatively simple bureaucracies which in many cases merely paralleled the nursing hierarchies through which they had risen to institutional responsibility.[26]

Particularly in the larger and more bureaucratically complex hospitals, superintendents professionalizing their craft and marking out spheres of authority had to contend with power wielded by others who already played important roles in the hospital. Notable in this regard were the trustees. They had created the superintendency, delegating authority to a steward or caretaker they hired and over whom they exercised oversight. Superintendents derived their power from the trustees; they owed deference in return. It was not uncommon for lay superintendents especially to share their trustees' world view and notions of the hospital as a moral universe rather than a bureaucratic organization. This complex relationship showed strains as superintendents tried to function more as executives and less as caretakers. Even George H.M. Rowe, who enjoyed exceptionally good rapport with the governing board of his Boston City Hospital, felt the need to point out that a superintendent functioned most effectively when vested with executive authority. In other discussions, one can sometimes detect a pained embarrassment at the low esteem in which trustee boards sometimes held their superintendents. J.T. Duryea complained in his presidential address, for example, that trustees sometimes perceived 'night watchmen or other accidents of employment' as suitable superintendents.[27] The superintendent's chief advantage in expanding his role and his authority *vis à vis* his superiors stemmed from his mastery of institutional detail that left even the most intensely involved trustee dependent on him.[28]

Superintendents were more successful in asserting leadership over their fellow servants within the hospital. Like other nineteenth-century employers, hospitals drew many of their employees – housekeepers, ward attendants, kitchen help, laundresses, and labourers – from a workforce not accustomed to the discipline required in increasingly complex institutions. Association sessions devoted considerable attention to administrative techniques for imposing order on the staff. Clocks, schedules, rules, record-keeping requirements, and printed forms routinized work, leaving ever less to the judgement of individual employees and putting ever more of the institution under bureaucratic control.[29] Even race could be an effective instrument for extending the superintendent's authority; Dr Eugene Elder of the Macon (Georgia) Hospital commended black employees to his fellow superintendents because they were especially easy to control.[30]

Doctors proved the most enduring challenge to hospital administrators. Superintendents based their aspirations to professional status on technical competence and the mastery of a body of arcane knowledge. But the claims of physicians clearly had widespread acceptance; the early twentieth-century reform of medical education, with its increasing emphasis on modern science, extended this advantage. These same changes in medical schooling would, by restricting access to the medical profession and thereby raising the social class origins of practitioners, broaden as well the social superiority that most hospital physicians enjoyed over their administrative counterparts. But it was to the age-old content of medical practice – the almost priestly role of explaining disease and reassuring the sick – that doctors most owed their advantaged position in the culture generally and in the hospital particularly.[31] Superintendents would find it difficult to interpose administrative edicts between doctor and patient.

Only the most eccentric superintendents publicly questioned the autonomy of physicians, but the problem of controlling the medical staff was a frequent undercurrent in Association proceedings.[32] The often-repeated debate over whether superintendents needed to be medically qualified generally returned to the same issue: Would doctor-administrators be better able than laymen to secure the co-operation of hospital physicians?[33] It is tempting to see the conflict between doctors and superintendents over the latter's control of institutional discipline and costs in terms of the professional aspirations of administrators. But the superintendents should not be understood solely as advocates of a modern hospital bureaucracy. Rather, many of them very much remained representatives of the more traditional views of the trustees, speaking as voices from the past against the interest of physicians in transforming the hospital into a modern medical workshop. Superintendents articulated lay concerns that doctors sometimes cared more about disease than about their patients. They were sensitive to the careerism – both intellectual and financial – that physicians sometimes brought into the hospital. And some superintendents expressed reservations about tying the fortunes of hospitals and their patients too closely to the modern teaching and research agendas of medical schools. Yet it was ordinarily only when they spoke for the trustees that most early twentieth-century superintendents could hope to prevail in these clashes of values with physicians.[34]

It was not until the late twentieth-century transformation of third-party payment that the balance of power within the hospital began to shift noticeably from physicians to administrators. Neither the workmen's compensation programmes introduced in the 1910s nor the Blue Cross-Blue Shield plans that began in the 1930s and expanded greatly in the postwar decades significantly altered the internal organization of the hospital. It had indeed been the intent of the Blue Cross system to preserve the institution precisely as it existed.[35] Likewise, the Medicare and Medicaid reforms of the great society were expected to leave the hospital structurally unchanged while making medical treatment more broadly available. But government assumption of responsibility for the health care for millions of elderly and poor Americans led ultimately to substantial change in the health care system.[36]

Massive federal funding channelled through programmes for patient care financed the development and acquisition of expensive new medical technologies, raising expectations and costs throughout the system. The same federal money underwrote dramatic increases in physicians' incomes.[37] An increasing reliance on complex technologies – often operated by non-physicians – further distanced relationships between practitioners and patients. The new level of physicians' incomes did the same. The inflow of federal money would ultimately undermine the cultural authority of doctors by dividing them from those they treated. At the same time, the hospitals in which they practised came ever more under the scrutiny of government officials concerned with what some feared to be costs rising inexorably toward national economic disaster. Regulations imposed by these outside authorities and administered by hospital managers seemed, by the mid-1980s, to be bringing the practice of hospital medicine under bureaucratic control. Doctors – no longer as able as before to argue that their opposition to reform derived from a principled commitment to patient care – were handicapped in resisting the intrusion of cost control and accountability. Joining their managerial colleagues in other areas of late-twentieth-century economic and institutional life, hospital administrators were able to proclaim the triumph of management. It was a victory in a quest not even imagined when their predecessors had embarked on the road to professionalization early in the twentieth century.

Notes

1. The standard histories of the American general hospital are Morris J. Vogel, *The Invention of the Modern Hospital: Boston, 1870–1930* (University of Chicago Press, Chicago, 1980) and Charles E. Rosenberg, *The Care of Strangers: The Rise of America's Hospital System* (Basic Books, New York, 1987).

2. The usually-cited figure of 178 hospitals in 1873 is in J.M. Toner, 'Statistics of regular medical associations and hospitals of the United States', *Transactions of the American Medical Association*, 24 (1873), 314–33. Toner's list includes fifty-eight institutions identifiable as insane asylums. Edwin H.L. Corwin, *The American Hospital* (Commonwealth Fund, New York, 1946) and Commission on Hospital Care, *Hospital Care in the United States* (Commonwealth Fund, New York, 1947) provide a wealth of data about the institution in the first half of the twentieth century.

3. Vogel, *Modern Hospital, passim*; Rosenberg, *Care of Strangers, passim*.

4. 'Association of Hospital Superintendents, report of the proceedings', *National Hospital and Sanitarium Record*, 3 (September, 1899), 1–3. Summary listings of the Association's first thirty-eight meetings can be found in Bert W. Caldwell, 'American Hospital Association', *American and Canadian Hospitals* (Physicians' Record Company, Chicago, 1937), 11–35. See also Alejandra C. Laszlo, 'The American Hospital Association: emergence of a professional organization, 1899–1914', unpublished paper, Department of History and Sociology of Science, University of Pennsylvania, January, 1986.

5. Within its first year of publication, Sutton shifted the *National Hospital and Sanitarium Record* from its complete identification with a convalescent food to a new product. The journal began to advocate uniform systems of hospital accounting and record-keeping and to carry editorials, endorsements, and advertising for preprinted forms and filing systems designed specifically for hospital use. See, for example, the December 1897, and the February and May 1898 issues in volume 1. Sutton later chronicled his success as a publisher of hospital forms in 'Past, present and future', *The International Hospital Record*, 15 (March, 1912), 7. Sutton sold the *International Hospital Record* to the American Hospital Association, reportedly because he 'found the work too exacting . . . especially in conjunction with his printing business and the publication of his system of hospital records': editorial, 'Announcement of purchase', *The Modern Hospital*, 4 (March, 1915), 183.

6. The *National Hospital and Sanitarium Record* evidently carried the only contemporaneous data for the first three meetings of the Association. See 3 (September, 1899), 1–3; 3 (August, 1900), 33–5; 5 (September, 1901), 3–9. The Association began to publish annual

accounts of its meetings – including lists of those attending – with its fourth annual conference in 1902. Titles vary, and the only original copy of the 1903 volume known to exist – *Proceedings of the Association of Hospital Superintendents of the United States and Canada* (hence *Proceedings AHA*) – is in the Countway Library of Harvard Medical School, Boston, Massachusetts.

7. For the general phenomenon of middle-class occupational organizations, see Robert H. Wiebe, *The Search for Order, 1877–1920* (Hill & Wang, New York, 1967), especially Chapter 5, 'A new middle class', 111–32. For scientific societies, see Margaret W. Rossiter, *Women Scientists in America: Struggles and Strategies to 1940* (Johns Hopkins University Press, Baltimore, 1982), 72–99. Burton J. Bledstein, *The Culture of Professionalism: The Middle Class and the Development of Higher Education in America* (Norton, New York, 1976).

8. Charles E. Rosenberg, 'And heal the sick: hospital and patient in 19th-century America', *Journal of Social History*, 10 (1977), 429–47, especially 437; William H. Williams, *America's First Hospital: The Pennsylvania Hospital, 1751–1841* (Haverford House, Wayne, PA, 1976), 52–4, 110–11, 140–2.

9. Responses from other institutions to an 1894 letter from the Massachusetts General Hospital asking about facilities for middle-class patients are in the Massachusetts General Archives, Private Ward (1894) folder, Phillips House file. On practices in Boston, F.A. Washburn and W.B. Howland, 'The training of hospital administrators', *Transactions of the American Hospital Association* (hence *Trans. AHA*), *12th Annual Conference* (hence *AC*), *1910*, 249–56; on New York, S.S. Goldwater, comment in minutes of the annual meeting, *Trans AHA, 8th AC, 1906*, 43.

10. For the perspective that physicians embracing scientific management brought to their parallel quest, see Ernest Amory Codman's memoir of his efforts to establish the American College of Surgeons in his text, *The Shoulder* (Thomas Todd Company, Boston, 1934), v–xi; epilogue, 1–29. Also Susan Reverby, 'Stealing the golden eggs: Ernest Amory Codman and the science and management of medicine', *Bulletin of the History of Medicine*, 55 (1981), 156–71; J.M.T. Finney, 'The standardization of the surgeon', *Journal of the American Medical Association*, 63 (1914), 1,433–7.

11. Examples include: C.S. Howell, 'Hospital construction', Frank E. Baker, 'Hospital ventilation', and ensuing discussion, all in *Proceedings AHA, 4th AC, 1902*, 141–7, 155–63; A.B. Ancker, 'Notes of the requirements of modern hospital architecture', Frank Miles Day, 'Hospital Architecture', and Henry M. Hurd, 'Modern hospital architecture: the pavilion hospital', *Trans AHA, 5th AC, 1903*, 81–128; Edmund Wheelwright, 'Hospital operating rooms and their accessories', Bertrand E. Taylor, 'The standardizing of hospital construction and equipment', and ensuing discussion, *Trans AHA, 7th AC, 1905*, 77–109. Superintendent (and later AHA

president) Thomas Howell attributed many of the increased costs to extravagance, asking rhetorically if hospitals were over-indulging their mostly poor patients with too much architectural ornament, and wondering whether the institutions were too quick to embrace medical fads like tiled surfaces to promote asepsis; Howell, 'Is the increased expenditure in hospital construction and equipment justified?' *Trans AHA, 7th AC, 1905*, 133–45.

12. J.A. Washburn, 'Medical organization and medical education in general hospitals', E.S. Gilmore, 'The organization of a teaching hospital', and ensuing discussion, *Trans AHA, 9th AC, 1907*, 131–46; Joseph Howland, 'Report of sub-committee on medical organization and medical education', *Trans AHA, 10th AC, 1908*, 353–5.

13. A.S. Kavanagh, 'Hospital support, and how to secure it', and ensuing discussion, *Trans AHA, 9th AC, 1907*, 64–78, 88–91. See also Vogel, *Modern Hospital*, 125–6.

14. C. Irving Fisher, 'Private patients in general hospitals', and ensuing discussion, *Trans AHA, 6th AC, 1904*, 93–104; George H.M. Rowe, 'Presidential Address', *Trans AHA, 7th AC, 1905*, 53–66, especially 57; Louis Curtis, 'The modern hotel-hospital', *Trans AHA, 9th AC, 1907*, 182–8. Thomas Howell, Superintendent of New York Hospital noted that

> very few managers of hospitals which maintain private patient services know whether they are conducting them at a profit, or at a loss, for the reason that they do not insist upon an accurate system of accounting being introduced and maintained. (Howell, 'Cost accounting in hospitals', *Trans AHA, 11th AC, 1909*, 193–205, especially 195)

For the role of physicians in attracting paying patients, see David Rosner, *A Once Charitable Enterprise: Hospitals and Health Care in Brooklyn and New York, 1885–1915* (Cambridge University Press, 1982).

15. Jane Addams, 'The layman's view of hospital work among the poor', *Trans AHA, 9th AC, 1907* 57–63.

16. Examples include: John Peters, 'Dispensary abuse', *Proceedings AHA, 4th AC, 1902* 119–27; Franklin B. Kirkbride, 'Uses and abuses of dispensaries', *Proceedings AHA, 5th AC, 1903*, 172–85; R.R. Ross, 'Presidential address', *Trans AHA, 9th AC, 1907*, 50–6; John Peters, 'The development of the work and the restriction of the abuse of the out-patient department', and Thomas Howell, 'Method of investigating out-patient applicants at Worcester hospitals', both in *Trans AHA, 10th AC, 1908*, 268–73, 280–4.

17. Josephine E. Royan, 'Hospital housekeeping', M.W. M'Kechnie, 'Hospital housekeeping', Maud Banfield, 'The cleaning', and John Peters, 'Hospital dietary', all in *Proceedings AHA, 5th AC, 1903*, 45–80, 151–70; Renwick Ross, 'Artificial refrigeration',

and John H. McCollom, 'The destruction of refuse and disinfection', *Trans AHA, 7th AC, 1905* 209–38; M. Wahlstrom, 'Breakage and loss, and how far should employees be held responsible?' and William O. Mann, 'My experience with floors', *Trans AHA, 9th AC, 1907*, 99–111; John Hornsby, 'Some scientific aspects of hospital administration', *Trans AHA, 10th ACA, 1908*, 219–36.

18. J.T. Duryea, 'Annual address of the president', *Proceedings AHA, 4th AC, 1902*, 20–4.

19. F.A. Washburn, 'Some methods of utilizing hospital waste', Jeremiah Long, 'Engine room economies', and ensuing discussions, *Trans AHA, 7th AC, 1905*, 239–56; R.W. Bruce Smith, 'Waste in hospitals', *Trans AHA, 9th AC, 1907*, 147–54.

20. In his presidential address, Duryea called attention to the need for superintendents to establish an agreed-upon knowledge base:

> The troubles and trials of each of us have individualities not peculiar to all of us. We teach ourselves to meet and master the obstacles that we encounter, and the little crystals of wisdom and direction that come to us from these virtues are the jewels in our crown of rejoicing. In these instances, our methods are not our own, they should belong to all of us. We require them to be individually and mutually successful. We come to these conferences hungry and thirsty for ideas, intelligent, well digested ideas of management, of government, of finance, of construction, of training schools, of our boards, of each other, and we ask them from all of you. (*Proceedings AHA, 4th AC, 1902*, 20–4)

21. The impact of scientific management in the hospital is discussed in Charles E. Rosenberg, 'Inward vision and outward glance: the shaping of the American hospital, 1880–1914', *Bulletin of the History of Medicine*, 53 (1979), 346–91. The broader scientific management movement in the United States was particularly associated with engineer Frederick W. Taylor. One of his briefer explanations of 'Taylorism' is 'A piece-work system', *Transactions of the American Society of Mechanical Engineers*, 16 (1895), 856–903. Critical analyses are in Harry Braverman, *Labor and Monopoly Capital* (Monthly Review Press, New York, 1974), especially Chapter 5, 'The primary effects of scientific management', and David F. Noble, *America by Design: Science, Technology, and the Rise of Corporate Capitalism* (Knopf, New York, 1979).

22. The first issue of *Modern Hospital*, the Association's journal, appeared in 1913. A bibliography of works on hospital construction, management, and the like appeared in the conference proceedings in 1904, even before the publication of the first handbooks of hospital administration: Charlotte A. Aikens (ed.), *Hospital Management* (W.B. Saunders, Philadelphia, 1911); Albert J. Ochsner and

Meyer Strum, *The Organization, Construction and Management of Hospitals* (Cleveland Press, Chicago, 1909); and John Hornsby and Richard Schmidt, *The Modern Hospital* (W.B. Saunders, Philadelphia, 1913). Training emerged as a theme at superintendents' conventions in 1907 when members petitioned the Association to organize a two- or three-week summer course on hospital work. S.S. Goldwater reported to the same meeting, as chair of the Association's Committee on Hospital Progress, the establishment of a chair of hospital management and economics at the new Brooklyn Post-Graduate Medical School and the fact that a New York-area university – evidently Columbia University Teacher's College – was about to establish a department for training hospital superintendents:

> Thus approaches the realization of a hope long cherished by many members of the Association, that the technical training of hospital superintendents might be undertaken by an educational body of dignity, learning, foresight and influence, not for the greater glory of those who are already engaged in the labor of hospital administration, but for the greater efficiency and better social service of their successors. (*Trans AHA, 9th AC, 1907*, 46–7, 151–71)

The Massachusetts General Hospital developed two parallel educational programmes for administrators – a three- to four-month programme for alumni of the hospital's nursing school, and a several-year training rotation in which physicians served on the hospital staff as assistant directors – early in the twentieth century. Detroit's Grace Hospital had a programme for graduate nurses similar to that in Boston: F.A. Washburn and W.B. Howland, 'The training of hospital administrators', *Trans AHA, 12th AC, 1910*, 249--65. See also, Frederic A. Washburn, *The Massachusetts General Hospital: its Development, 1900–1935* (Houghton Mifflin, Boston, 1939), 27.

23. Superintendent Charlotte Aikens complained in 1906 that the Association of Hospital Superintendents was only a paper shell; annual meetings and rotating officers were inadequate to the organization's needs. Properly organized, a superintendents' association could not only promote learning and co-operation among its members, but it could also interpret its mandate more broadly and earn the trust of the public at the same time. A stronger Association could, for example, prevent the 'unnecessary duplication' of hospitals: 'Development of a wider national association', *Trans AHA, 8th AC, 1906*, 150–60, especially 157; Thomas Howell, 'Report of the committee on the development of the association', *Trans AHA, 10th AC, 1908*, 210–18. In 1913 the Association appointed a committee to study the possibility of a permanent headquarters and year-round organization – in part

because of the greater public good that such a reorganization could accomplish: E.P. Haworth, 'What the American Hospital Association can do for the hospitals of America' and ensuing discussion, *Trans AHA, 15th AC, 1913*, 256–73. The Association's first permanent headquarters opened in Philadelphia in 1917: Laszlo, 'American Hospital Association', 38. Professionalizers also realized that they had to earn the public trust by policing their own ranks. For one of the occasional admissions that some superintendents were not adequate to their tasks, see Duryea, 'Annual address of the president', *Proceedings AHA, 4th AC, 1902*, 23. Bledstein argues the link between claims to technical expertise and the exercise of cultural authority with particular vehemence: *Culture of Professionalism, passim.*

24. J.C. Biddle, 'The physician as a hospital superintendent', C.S. Howell, 'The layman as a superintendent', and ensuing discussion, *Trans AHA, 6th AC, 1904*, 47–53, 58–68.

25. See, for example, the presidential address of layman superintendent Daniel D. Test, *Trans AHA, 6th AC, 1904*, 43–6.

26. Membership lists, with professional degrees and institutional affiliations, are published in the annual transactions.

27. George H.M. Rowe, 'Observations on hospital administration', J.T. Duryea, 'Annual address of the president', both in *Proceedings AHA, 4th AC, 1902*, 51–67, 20–4.

28. Herbert B. Howard, long-time administrator of the Massachusetts General Hospital, reminded his peers that trustees depended for information on the superintendent, who has 'entire charge of the details of his institution': Howard, 'The managers and the superintendent', *Proceedings AHA, 4th AC, 1902*, 68–70.

29. See, for example, James B. Woodward, 'Hospital organization' with ensuing discussion, *Proceedings AHA, 4th AC, 1902*, 71–88; C. Irving Fisher, 'Uniformity in hospital financial reports and statistics' and ensuing discussion, *Trans AHA, 7th AC, 1905*, 257–82; R.H. Townley, 'Discipline and organization' and ensuing discussion, *Trans AHA, 8th AC, 1906*, 84–95; M. Wahlstrom, 'Breakage and loss, and how far should employees be held responsible?' and Asa Bacon, 'The selection and management of hospital employees: a comparison of hospital pay rolls', both in *Trans AHA, 9th AC, 1907*, 99–104, 112–19.

30. Eugene Elder, 'The management of the race question in hospitals', *Trans 9th AC, 1907* 127–30.

31. On the impact of reform in medical education on the social status of physicians, see Howard S. Berliner, 'A larger perspective on the Flexner Report', *International Journal of Health Services*, 5 (1975), 573–92; on the hieratic role of physicians, a good place to start is Charles E. Rosenberg, 'The therapeutic revolution: medicine, meaning, and social change in nineteenth-century America', in Morris J. Vogel and Charles E. Rosenberg (eds), *The Therapeutic Revolution: Essays in the Social History of American Medicine*

(University of Pennsylvania Press, Philadelphia, 1979), 3–25.

32. For example, Alice Seabrook, 'Appointment of internes' and ensuing discussion, *Trans AHA 8th AC, 1906* 195–200.

33. J.C. Biddle, 'The physician as hospital superintendent' and discussion, *Trans AHA, 6th AC, 1904*, 47–50, 58–68; Henry M. Hurd, 'The medical organization of hospitals' and discussion, *Trans AHA, 8th AC, 1906* 72–83.

34. George P. Ludlam, 'Presidential address', *Trans AHA, 8th AC, 1906*, 63–71.

35. On workmen's compensation, see Vogel, *Modern Hospital*, 121–4. On Blue Cross, Ronald L. Numbers, 'The third party: health insurance in America', in Vogel and Rosenberg (eds), *The Therapeutic Revolution*, 177–200, especially 182–3; and Rosemary Stevens, *American Medicine and the Public Interest* (Yale University Press, New Haven, 1971), 269–72.

36. Stevens, *American Medicine*, 444–527.

37. On increased expenditures, Numbers, 'Third party', 189; on physicians' incomes, Robert Stevens and Rosemary Stevens, *Welfare Medicine in America: A Case Study of Medicaid* (The Free Press, New York, 1974), 194.

Index